abounding health
naturally

Blessings!
Sharon Jean
III John 1:2

abounding health
naturally

Sharon Jean Wiginton

TATE PUBLISHING & *Enterprises*

Abounding Health Naturally
Copyright © 2010 by Sharon Jean Wiginton. All rights reserved.

No part of this publication may be reproduced, stored in a retrieval system or transmitted in any way by any means, electronic, mechanical, photocopy, recording or otherwise without the prior permission of the author except as provided by USA copyright law.

The opinions expressed by the author are not necessarily those of Tate Publishing, LLC.

Published by Tate Publishing & Enterprises, LLC
127 E. Trade Center Terrace | Mustang, Oklahoma 73064 USA
1.888.361.9473 | www.tatepublishing.com

Tate Publishing is committed to excellence in the publishing industry. The company reflects the philosophy established by the founders, based on Psalm 68:11,
"The Lord gave the word and great was the company of those who published it."

Book design copyright © 2010 by Tate Publishing, LLC. All rights reserved.
Cover design by Kristen Verser
Interior design by Stephanie Woloszyn

Published in the United States of America

ISBN: 978-1-61663-334-9
1. Health & Fitness / Food Content Guides
2. Health & Fitness / Diseases / General
10.05.24

acknowledgments

Thinking about all the people I would like to acknowledge and thank for the help they have been to me during this journey is overwhelming. God so blessed me with an army of friends and family who held me up when I was diagnosed with stage three breast cancer; friends and family who not only stood with me in prayer, but in giving me their time and encouragement. God's people certainly helped me get through this most difficult yet rewarding time in my life.

I had many friends who called me day after day who wanted to pray with me and to remind me of God's faithfulness. Some of these friends would call me just when I had breathed a prayer for God to send someone to encourage me. It was amazing how faithfully God answered those prayers with just the right people who had just the right things to say to pull me through that particular time. Thank you, each one of you, my precious friends. I am still in awe when I stop to think about those dark days in my life and how strong you were for me. Kathy, you and Lena called me many times to let me know you were not only praying for me, but fasting too. Many times when I couldn't pray for myself because I was so afraid, I remember Dawn would remind me, "It's okay, we are praying for you!" There were times when I wavered and doubted that nutrition would really help heal my body. During these times, Lena reminded me that I was made after God's own image, and my body would work the way He designed it to work. My dear friend, A.C. helped me learn to put all my thoughts through God's thought test in Philippians and prayed through much "wrong thinking" with me. The Philippians test still helps me to this day!

Thank you to my sweet family in Oklahoma! Not one of you doubted that I made the right choice by going the nutritional route to heal my body. Each of you was overjoyed that I turned away from traditional medicine and chose an "alternative" path. Your prayers for me and your confidence in the path I took meant so much to me.

To my children, I cannot begin to express my gratefulness to you and to the Lord *for* you. Kristin, you were already grown and away from home when I was diagnosed with cancer, but it was so touching to me to hear you say, "Why couldn't this have happened when I was still at home so I could help you?" That really meant a lot to me. I also want to thank you for the precious grandchildren you have given us. Our very first grandchild, Ethan, was born just a few days after the diagnosis. What a bright ray of light in such a dark time of my life. It makes me smile even now when I think how God gave us such a special gift at the perfect time. Kara, you were old enough to drive, so much of the burden of getting all the children where they needed to be fell on you. You worked hard to keep the house running when I just couldn't, and you did a great job in re-learning how to fix our meals! You were only sixteen, but you carried a heavy burden, and you did it with grace. Now you have a family of your own and have given us a beautiful granddaughter. I know God will bless you with His strength as you raise your own family. Johnny, Phillip, Jenna, and Patrick, you have walked the path with me and have been wonderful in all the changes we have made in our home. I know it has not been easy to eat so differently and it has, at times, made life a bit difficult for you. I know you have endured some teasing about being health nuts and about the weird carrot-greens juice you drink, but you have taken it so well and have proven to be strong and determined. I hope you take this knowledge of health with you when you begin your own family. It is so much easier to stay healthy than to have to regain lost health.

John, my wonderful husband—what can I say? You gave up night after night of sleep to read Scripture to me. You stayed home from work many days in a row because I couldn't let go of you. After the initial shock of the diagnosis wore off and we knew the path we wanted to take for my healing, you never doubted for a minute that I would be well. Not only that, you convinced me over and over that someday I would be helping others to understand true healing from the terrible disease of cancer. Thank you so much for believing in me, and thank you for loving me with unconditional love. Your voice still soothes me when I am anxious, and I love you more than I could ever express.

Dr. Robbins, thank you for sharing your knowledge of health with me. Thank you for your patience with me, and thank you for taking time to answer all my questions! I know the world has put you through much stress because of the stand you take, but I am so thankful you do not give up. You have taught and continue to teach me valuable lessons, and I am so grateful God prepared the path before me with a doctor such as you.

Thank you to the wonderful staff at Dr. Robbins's clinic. You are all jewels! I remember the first time I walked into the clinic I wanted to just pack my bags and park myself there until I was well! The warm, loving atmosphere was in stark contrast to the doctors' offices I had been in at the beginning of the cancer diagnosis. I came from offices where I felt a sadness and death sentence over me into such a bright, cheerful office where only hope and love were felt. Teri, I have never met a more patient woman in my life! I know for so long I called you not just once a day, but three and four times...even more than that on some days! You never once made me feel like a bother. You saw through to my fear and just loved me through it. To this day I know I can call you with concerns and questions. You showed such discernment and wisdom and steered me to align my thinking with Scripture. Michelle, I know you are not part of Dr. Robbins' staff, but you are the one who directed me to him. You are also the one who "slapped me around" when I needed it! There were times I needed to get my mind off my problems and quit feeling sorry for myself. You knew just how to help me do that! It didn't matter what time of day or night, you were (and still are!) always there for me.

Of course, most of all, I thank my precious Lord and Savior. I am so grateful to know that when my life on this earth is over, I will spend eternity with Him. Until then, I pray to have His *Abounding Health, Naturally!*

table of contents

foreword 11

introduction 13

looking back.. 19

my wake-up call…cancer 23

germs, germs everywhere! (who's responsible 29
for this mess?)

have we learned *anything* from history?............................. 39

the choice of health care 51

who really wants great health? 57

what is great health? 69

why we should eat for great health....................................... 75

what we should eat for great health 83

how to eat for great health 95

eating healthy on the go.. 105

what to expect in the beginning—cleaning up 113
the diet and detoxing

organic versus conventionally grown 119

healing from disease 123

the best of the best 141

live life in motion!.. 149

a merry heart does good... 155

faith in god and service to others 161

menu ideas and recipes 165

afterword 177

resources 179

foreword

When Sharon Jean Wiginton was diagnosed with cancer, who would have thought that God would use such a *terrible* occurrence to change her life—physically, attitudinally, and spiritually? God is an amazing God. No, He doesn't make all of our fairy tale dreams come true as we think they should, but He does use all that we experience, good or bad, for our good and for His glory. God does not allow us to suffer what we consider a bad thing just for drill. It is always with a purpose. Through the struggles and trials in life, we are all given many opportunities to grow and thus be more usable for our higher calling—furthering the kingdom. Unfortunately, most run from the classrooms and lessons that God prepares especially for us to prepare us to accomplish that for which we were created.

Sharon Jean, while initially frightened and scared (and who wouldn't be?) by her diagnosis of cancer, chose to use the trial to dig deeper, seek out uncommon truth, and find answers that God had provided from the beginning of creation. As a result, not only is she disease free and healthy, but she has been motivated to help and influence her husband, her family, and many friends to follow God's principles of physical and spiritual health. As if that were not enough, God saw to it that she author this most practical and inspiring work.

The information in this book is life changing. It

contains God's pearls of truth relative to preventing and reversing disease. It is a book written from the heart, from a changed life, that of Sharon Jean.

When I think of what cancer did to produce this tremendous work, one of my favorite quotes comes to mind:

A message prepared in the mind reaches other minds.
A message prepared in the heart reaches other hearts;
But a message prepared in a life reaches other lives.

Sharon Jean's *Abounding Health, Naturally!* is a message prepared in a life—hers.

—Joel Robbins, D.C., N.D., M.D.

introduction

I have wanted for some time to write a book on nutrition and health. Over the last few years, my husband and others, from close friends to cashiers at the grocery store, have been telling me, "You should write a book." It probably sounds funny that strangers would be suggesting I write a book on health, but when our grocery carts are full of raw fruits and vegetables, we tend to draw the attention of those around us. People want to know why we buy so much fresh produce and ask questions like, "How can you use it all before it spoils?" From one question to another, invariably a conversation starts about nutrition. I usually get around to why we personally started eating mostly fresh and raw fruits and vegetables, and by then people are hooked on wanting to know more.

I have been invited to give talks on nutrition and how it relates to our health, and each time I was encouraged by people I didn't even know, "You should write a book." I have also spent hours and hours on the phone with people who want to understand more about nutrition. Sometimes my husband could hear these phone conversations I had and he'd gently remind me, "Honey, you need to write your book."

I thought long and hard about writing on nutrition. Several times I did start writing, only to put it aside for months. While I always love talking to people about the difference proper nutrition can make in our lives, I wasn't sure I was the one who should write a book on the topic. I kept thinking and even saying to my husband, "Who am I...what do I know that isn't common knowledge?" I honestly did not realize how much I have learned over the last several years, and I did not see that most people do not understand that the way we eat directly affects our health and vitality.

As I thought about all the different people who have asked me for information and advice, I began to put together what it was they wanted. They wanted hope; hope that they or their loved ones could find healing from illness and disease. They truly wanted to understand how to eat and feed their families so that they could live healthy lives without fear of the diseases that seem to be "common" to every family in one way or another.

The information available from the medical community does not offer any real hope. Most doctors can only give us help in living *with* a disease or illness, not help in completely healing and living with vibrancy, free from aches and pains.

This is one thing I have thought so much about when I pondered writing. I wanted to share with many people the hope, actually the assurance that God made our bodies to live in health. As my doctor, Dr. Joel Robbins, taught me, "Health is a gift; disease is something you earn." I wanted people to understand that it is their responsibility to not only gain health, but to live in health. I realized they cannot do that unless they have the knowledge they need to make healthy choices.

In making these choices about health and in looking for information, you must exercise caution. There are all kind of books and articles wanting to tell you what proper nutrition is. The Internet is full of varying opinions on what healthy eating looks like. Pray for God to give you great discernment as you begin to educate yourself. I can heartily recommend all of Dr. Joel Robbins' materials on health and nutrition, but even he says in his teachings, "Don't make me your authority. Just listen to what I have to say and see if it makes sense to you." So as you read, study, and listen to people speak about health, do so with your mind and your spirit.

Much information is readily available to us about the value raw foods are to our bodies. A big problem is the information is mostly presented in such a way that causes many Christians to shun it. People who call themselves "raw foodists" are taking the major lead in turning people on to eating food as it is grown in nature. While much of the information they are giving is correct, the style with which they are delivering it is wrong. God is not getting the credit He deserves in creating our bodies to be in health. He is the One who designed the perfect diet for us from the very beginning. It was all His idea, His creation.

It has made me very sad to see these "raw foodists" take the truth and pervert it enough that God-fearing Christians want no part of it. Think about it though. No group of people no matter how "spiritually enlightened" they are have the ability or the intelligence to think up such an amazing design for our body. God designed our bodies to be in health and to be self-healing, but only when we treat them the way He prescribed!

Dr. Robbins once told me, "Remember that truth is truth, and God is the author and creator of all truth. Satan has not created anything; he has only perverted what God has made. Even the new age people have nuggets of truth in their teachings. The problem is their motive for using that truth is self-serving, as opposed to using it to serve God. A truth taught by a cult does not make it falsehood. To disregard God's truth simply because you heard it from some cult would be the same as saying because certain cults use the Bible, we now must stop reading it."

One happening in particular that woke me up to this problem was when Dr. Robbins was invited to a biblical health seminar to speak on nutrition. When the head of the seminar got Dr. Robbins' notes and saw the teaching was on raw food, he called Dr. Robbins and said, "No, just come and speak on attitudes and health instead." I talked with this man's personal assistant, and he told me, "Sharon, you just do not know how many times we have been stung by raw foodists." I tried to tell him that Dr. Robbins' teachings are nothing like that. I told him that I understood exactly what he meant, but that these teachings are very biblically based and sound. The head of the conference held firm that year, though, that Dr. Robbins would just come and speak on attitudes. Dr. Robbins very graciously went, and I believe those in leadership there must have seen his heart because the next year he was invited back to speak on nutrition!

Through this book and in seminars and teachings, I hope to shed light on some lies we have believed about our health. I hope to share a vision; a vision for living a life pleasing to the Lord. Even though I used nutrition to heal from cancer, I want more than that now. I want to live my life, until the day I die, serving others and the Lord. I can only do that when I am healthy and energetic.

I have a responsibility to take care of this temple God has given me and to live out this earthly life in a way that is pleasing to Him.

It is not enough to just want to heal from illness and disease. We must gain knowledge and then take responsibility for how we live. We need to make choices that will allow us to live in health. For the most part, we do not take time to gain the knowledge we need until we understand our need for the knowledge. I hope through this book you will see your need for knowledge in what our bodies require to stay in health. I pray this book will be the beginning of your own journey to health and maybe even the start of your quest for knowledge in how God made our bodies to live in health.

looking back

While I definitely identify with the thoughts behind *I just want to get well*, we need to understand this thinking is simply not enough. I have seen from people I have known and loved personally that it is not enough to just get well. You must somehow get a vision for living your life in health. You must gain knowledge and educate yourself on how to live a healthy life pleasing to God.

I have known people who have been healed completely from cancer by changing their diet and lifestyle, only to return to their old eating habits and then have cancer return in their body. It wasn't that the cancer was not really gone.... it was. Cancer, though, can return quickly when the environment in the body goes back to what caused it in the first place. Many of these people just could not fully understand the connection between diet and cancer and never fully committed themselves to this new lifestyle. As I grieved over these people and wondered, "What went wrong?" each time I came up with generally the same answer. Not one of these people actually got to the point where they educated themselves on health. They had only listened to advice on how to gain their health again, but it didn't become a way of life to them. They didn't fully understand the role that nutrition, joyful gratefulness, and faith in God have in our health. Some of these people remained in such fear of the diagnosis that they could not fully recover. Fear and faulty thinking takes a huge toll on the body. Wrong thinking will consume much of the body's energy that no amount of healthy eating can replace.

I do understand how fear can overpower your thinking. When I was diagnosed with cancer, I was terrified. In light of what we are told about cancer (and other diseases), it is understandable. From the information we are given, it would seem that we have no power at all over disease. Illness and disease just "creep up" on you and one day you find yourself sick with no real hope. Who wouldn't be afraid of being diagnosed with cancer when the only answers are the ones the medical community has to offer? When you are able to get rid of that fear and faulty thinking through knowledge, you are arming yourself with the truth about health, and you have the ability to make wise choices and live in confidence and peace.

A big roadblock in gaining knowledge about health is apathy. Face it: most of us just do not care enough to read and study about nutrition. We would rather not know the effect the food we are eating is having on our bodies. It is not until we are faced with a health crisis that we wake up and begin to question what is going wrong with our bodies. Even when faced with such a crisis, some people let others make all the health care decisions for them. So much of the time we'd rather not take responsibility for our own health. It is much easier to go to the doctor and let him tell us what we need to do.

That was the story of *my* journey to health. I look back now and see I was on the ignorance and apathy road for all of my "before cancer" life. As a young adult, I had one health problem after another, yet I never stopped to try to understand why my body was struggling with one "minor" thing after another. I let the doctors take responsibility for my health and followed blindly what they said I needed to do. I think I knew nutrition was important, but I didn't care enough to truly understand and make the changes needed.

My earliest memories of real problems with my health go back to my late teens. My husband and I married when I was only eighteen, and we decided we wanted children right away. Year after year went by with disappointment after disappointment. Finally after five years of marriage, I went to a specialist who did surgery and "corrected" my problem. Very soon after that surgery, I conceived our first child. Several more years went by and eventually I had another surgery for infertility. Another problem was "corrected," and I was able to conceive our second child. Life went on, and God did choose to give us four more children with no medical intervention.

Little did I know at the time, though, that there were things very wrong within my body. I had many signs that things were not right, but I never caught on to these clues. At least some of these clues should have been very obvious. I lived most of my married life struggling with weight issues and at times, severe depression. Then, when our fifth child was a bit over a year old, I had surgery for a fibroid tumor on a gland behind my ear. Several years later, after we had our sixth child, I suffered four miscarriages, each a year and a half apart.

Through all this suffering, I never stopped to understand what was going on inside my body. I never questioned why I had so many health problems. Even when I had a huge fibroid tumor in my uterus and had a hysterectomy, I did not question the advice I was being given.

I, of all people, should never judge anyone who has health problems and does not take responsibility for them. Still, I find myself doing that very thing. I find myself so frustrated when it seems like people just do not care enough about their health to change their lifestyle, yet I was once one of those very people.

The path I chose was apathy and ignorance when it came to my health. That path was about to change drastically.

February 13, 2004, was the date of my wake-up call.

my wake-up call...cancer

I can remember all the way back to my childhood stories of people who were living and dying with cancer. Most people lived in dread of what is called "the big C," and I was one of them. That seemed to be the ultimate fear for most people.

When someone you knew got that diagnosis, you looked at them differently. They were now part of that group of people who "have cancer." Even if their treatment for cancer went well, you wondered if someday you'd hear they have cancer again...usually this time, much worse. We looked at these people expecting them to have cancer again any day; fully expecting to hear they were suffering through the treatments for cancer again. These people more often than not eventually died.

Then when it was I who was on the other end of the diagnosis, I was suddenly one of these people. I even viewed myself differently. I stayed in extreme fear for months. I could not get the words of the oncologist out of my mind, "If you do not do as I say and take chemo and radiation, you will be dead in six months. If you do what I say, you may live five or ten years."

I did not understand then that the traditional medical doctors do not have the answer for cancer, partly because they do not even know themselves what the disease is or how it happens. It just happens.

My husband and I prayed and begged God to show us what to do. My husband made the remark that he sure wanted me around more than just the five or ten years that the oncologist assured me of *if* I would do things his way.

I began to think about what I did know about cancer. I had read a book about nutritional healing from cancer many years before and told myself, "If I ever got cancer, this is what I would do." Isn't it sad that I didn't understand I didn't have to wait for that diagnosis? I could change the way I lived my life and never have to worry about that "if." I am grateful that I read that book because when the time came that I did indeed get cancer, I knew what I wanted to do. I just did not know how to do it.

In the midst of our turmoil, a friend called and told me about another friend whose sister went to a doctor who taught nutrition and she was healed of breast cancer. She encouraged me to call this friend. I did, and I got my first ray of encouragement! She was so lighthearted about my diagnosis and said, "Oh, you'll be fine! Just call Dr. Robbins and get started."

This lighthearted attitude was in such contrast to the demeanor other people had when they found out I was diagnosed, and it did much to begin turning my thinking around. This friend, along with a few others in my life, became lifelines of hope to me when I felt desperate. I somehow knew I had to change the way I was thinking about myself, along with learning about nutrition.

Actually, I did not start out to "learn" about nutrition. I only wanted to know what to do to get well. I soon understood that I had to learn, to dig, and to gain all the knowledge I could about cancer and the role nutrition plays in healing from cancer. It was also important to me that I gain assurance that I would not spend the rest of my life worrying about cancer reoccurring in my body.

I spent hours at a time doing all the reading I could. I listened to Dr. Robbins' audio tapes on health and nutrition and watched his teaching videos over and over. When I went to his office for a visit, I would buy another of his audio tapes to listen to on the drive home. I also found resources on the Internet about cancer and nutritional healing. I prayed for wisdom and discernment and God led me to the knowledge I needed.

The more I learned the more enthusiasm I had to keep learning. At times, though, I felt very frustrated. I wanted so badly for other people to know and understand the things I knew. I learned from Phillip Day of Credence that cancer is a healing process that has not been able to stop. Cancer begins wherever the body is being damaged. The trophoblast cells, those cells in the body designed by our Creator to heal, go to do their job. On completion of that job, we have enzymes that "turn off" the healing process (*Cancer, the Winnable War*).

When the body has been fueled for years on mostly lifeless food, then there is not available to the body the ability to turn the healing process off. A tumor or cancer mass then develops. In essence, cancer is a healing process gone awry.

As I began to learn this, a light came on! It all made so much sense! Why didn't everyone know this? Think about it. When you hear the statement, "Smoking causes cancer," change that thought to "Smoking causes damage to the lungs, the healing cells go to heal the damage, the healing cannot be turned off because of nutritional deficiencies in the body, and cancer develops." It's a mouthful, I realize that, but it is important to change the way you think about cancer…and any disease for that matter.

The same thing can be said of any cancer. It does not matter where the cancer begins; it always begins as a healing process because of damage to the body. When you hear of environmental pollutants that "cause cancer" change your thinking to "those things are damaging the body. Then the body does what our Creator designed it to do; it sends healing cells. If the body is not nutritionally sound enough to be able to turn off the healing process, cancer then begins."

It almost sounds too easy, but know this: it only seems that way because we have been taught that cancer is a mysterious disease that happens to some people. In reality, it will happen to most people at some point in their lives unless we make a change. We are seeing that in the rising cancer statistics.

Think of hundreds of years ago when scurvy was believed to be a mysterious disease that could possibly even be genetic. As authorities looked for causes of scurvy they saw how fathers went to sea, got scurvy and died. Their sons went to sea, got scurvy and died. "Ah!" They thought, "Scurvy must be genetic!" For years and years, thousands of people died of scurvy. This was mostly because the authorities were too stubborn to believe it could be a vitamin deficiency. That was just too simple of an explanation. We now see no one suffering from scurvy, and we would laugh if we knew someone was afraid of contracting scurvy. "It's all so simple," we'd say, "just make sure to get vitamin C in your diet!"

So, in the case of cancer, as Phillip Day says in his audio, *Cancer, the Winnable War*, "Science has done what science was supposed to do." Science showed many years ago what cancer is; the answer just has never made it out to the general public. He also states in his book, *Cancer, Why We're Still Dying to Know the Truth*, "Can we beat cancer? Yes. It's already done. The knowledge to conquer cancer was understood many decades ago, yet tragically the facts have not made it into the public domain until relatively recently." I can only think of one reason this information is not made widely known. As I listened to Phillip Day tell how the American Cancer Association is the most profitable nonprofit organization in the world and how "there are more people making a living from cancer than are dying from it," it became very clear why this life-saving information is not getting out to the public.

I know it sounds like a conspiracy theory and may even be just too hard for most people to believe. It is difficult to think about the millions of people who have gone through the ravages of chemotherapy and radiation, only to hear now that the answer is as simple as nutrition. It's a hard thing for me to say because I know how potentially painful this information can be; how devastating to think someone we know and loved suffered needlessly at the hands of medical science.

I did have two lumpectomies after the initial diagnosis. Because cancer was found in over half of the lymph nodes, it was placed at stage three breast cancer. Even before the first surgery, I started with a change in my diet. Since I knew from the beginning I did not want to go through chemotherapy and radiation, I knew I had to find other answers.

Just a little over two months after changing my diet, I found out that I was cancer free. Since I spent all that time also studying and reading about health, I knew I could never go back to my old ways and habits. I knew my whole lifestyle had changed for good!

germs, germs everywhere!
(who's responsible for this mess?)

I focused on cancer in the previous chapter because that was my story. That's the area I studied and learned about so I could be free from the fear of cancer. Cancer is the disease I think we fear the most and the disease that seems to be quickly advancing to the number one killer in our country.

The story is much the same, though, with any disease. We are not giving our body the nutrients it needs to continue to build healthy cells. The answer to disease is not found in the pharmaceuticals that are overtaking our country. People are finding themselves on more and more prescription medication with each passing year. Is that really the answer?

Are our bodies sick and tired because we have a lack of something that is in these chemicals? Of course not! These chemicals only work on the symptoms we are having, much like turning off the smoke detector instead of finding where and why the fire is burning and putting it out!

Let's begin to look closely at the commonly held beliefs most people have about health care. Does it make sense that prescription after prescription holds the only answers to our health problems? Prescription medication never solves any crisis going on in the body. They only quiet the symptoms. In reality, they stop the body's cry for help.

I briefly stated in the last chapter how the errors in the way people thought about scurvy actually cost thousands of lives. In this chapter and the next, I want to talk more in detail about "the germ theory" and the history of scurvy and other diseases that plagued so many people. Through this, I hope to show how changing the way we think about illness and disease can be the difference in life and death... to many, many people.

I talk much in this book about our responsibility in the matter of our health. I discussed in the very beginning of this book how important it is to educate yourself and fully understand your role in keeping your body healthy. I have already said that the way we think about illness and disease will affect not only you, but most everyone around you. The choices you make affect many people, especially the people in your own family.

If this is all true, if we are the ones responsible for how we age, whether we live out our lives in true health and whether our children will enjoy vibrant health, then what do germs have to do with it? If there are germs all around us, just waiting to infect us and make us sick, then how can we be responsible for staying healthy?

God says in His Word, in 1 Corinthians 6:19–20, "What? Know you not that your body is the temple of the Holy Ghost which is in you, which you have of God, and you are not your own? For you are bought with a price: therefore glorify God in your body, and in your spirit, which are God's." Since our body belongs to God in the same way our spirit belongs to Him, shouldn't we be honoring Him in our body and paying attention to our physical welfare just as we pay attention to our spiritual welfare?

If God created our bodies to be in health, and if He made a way for us to stay healthy by eating the food He created and thinking the thoughts He commanded, then why do we need immunizations, antibiotics, and a host of other things designed to ward off germs? It would seem that if that *were* true; if we do need all these chemicals in our body to make it function the way it should to stay in health, then did God miss something? Did He forget to plan for the onslaught of germs against our body?

Of course, the answer is no. God created our bodies to be miraculous, self-healing bodies. He gave us everything we need to stay healthy. He created the perfect food for us; He designed hard work for us to keep our bodies strong for the tasks He has before us. Our bodies were meant to last a lifetime, but that does not mean we can go about our way without regard to what our bodies need to be in health.

The laws God put into place regarding the health of our bodies work whether we know them or not. We may not know that the body has to have living foods to be able to make new living cells. It doesn't matter. Maybe we do not know that all the processed foods are toxic and causing us to fall into ill health, and the fast foods we consume day after day are pulling vital minerals from our bones and weakening them. Maybe some of us *do* know these things, but we just do not care. It doesn't matter. The law is in place and works whether we know it or not, whether we care or not.

It is much like gravity is in place and works whether someone knows about the law or not. One person may step off the edge of a tall building not knowing that gravity will pull him to the ground. Another person may step off that same edge knowing full well he will plummet to the ground because of gravity. It does not matter; their fate is the same.

So, the fact is: God created our bodies to be in health. He gave us the gift of health; we create disease and illness in our bodies by the choices we make. The germ theory is just one of many things man tries to buy in to so he will not be responsible. It is just another way to be able to live our lives without having to answer for the poor choices made.

The germ theory states that infectious diseases are caused by the activity of microorganisms within the body. In the medical schools of the United States and most other Western countries, doctors are taught about disease through the viewpoint of the germ theory. The scientist credited for discovering the germ theory is Louis Pasteur.

Louis Pasteur and a contemporary of his, Antoine Beauchamp, did much in the area of experimenting with the process of fermentation. These men were at the forefront in their fields of science.

Pasteur strongly believed and taught that we live in a hostile environment where germs were always trying to invade our bodies. His attitude was to protect the body from the harmful bacteria.

Beauchamp's teachings were completely the opposite. He believed that a healthy body would be immune to harmful bacteria and that only when the cells became weak could the bacteria cause an ill effect. Beauchamp's studies discovered that healthy tissue was always being exposed to bacteria, but that the germs are opportunistic and wait for the right conditions to thrive and grow. Those right conditions happen when our bodies are not fed properly and become run down and weakened.

Another prominent figure in those times was Claude Bernard. Bernard was France's leading physiologist and is considered the founder of experimental medicine. Where Pasteur believed the germ was everything, Bernard believed the terrain was the important factor in disease. Both men recognized the presence of microorganisms, but they differed greatly in how they viewed them. Pasteur was convinced they invaded the body from the outside, and Bernard was sure the inside of the body was first the problem.

On Pasteur's deathbed, with Claude Bernard present, Pasteur said, "Bernard avait raison. Le germ n'est rien, c'est le terrain qui est tout." This means, "Bernard was right, the seed is nothing. The soil is everything." It is interesting that Pasteur acknowledged Bernard instead of Beauchamp, when Beauchamp was the man he had been locked in a struggle with for decades.

An interesting analogy Beauchamp used to try and convince Pasteur of the error in the germ theory is about the relationship of flies to garbage. Would we say that flies create garbage? Or are the flies drawn to the existing garbage? Of course flies are drawn to the garbage! Flies are scavengers and they feed off of decaying matter. The association germs (flies) have with diseased tissue (garbage) is this: germs do not make the tissue weak, but the germs are drawn to the weak tissue.

Whether or not we get sick does not have so much to do with what germ we may catch, but really has more to do with whether we keep our bodies free of decaying matter that germs will be drawn to and feed on. The decaying matter these germs feed on is caused by poor nutrition and an unbalanced life.

Most of the germs that enter our bodies from the outside are quickly killed by our immune system. The microorganisms that live in our bodies and cause us to get sick can cause the illness because we provide them with a rich growth medium (the garbage) that they can feed on and then change into deadly bacteria, fungus, and viruses.

Let's get to the real reason we are experiencing so much illness and disease. Let's do the hard thing and take full responsibility for our health and the future health of our children and grandchildren.

Ask God to open your eyes and minds to the possibility that maybe, just maybe we have not understood the truth. This truth does not refer to just diseases, but even to the "everyday cold" and other illnesses that so hamper the way we live our lives.

Some amazing quotes to ponder:

> When we meet a fact which contradicts a prevailing theory, we must accept the fact and abandon the theory, even when the theory is supported by great names and is generally accepted.
> —Claude Bernard

> Had it not been for the mass selling of vaccines, Pasteur's germ theory would have collapsed into obscurity.
> —E. Douglas Hume
> ("Beauchamp or Pasteur?" 1932)

There is but one cause of disease, poison toxemia, most of which is created in the body by faulty living habits and faulty elimination

—Sir A. Lane (early 1900's)

It is time to lay to rest the notion that germs jump into people and cause diseases.

—Emanuel D., D.M.D.
(*Vitamin C: Who Needs It?* 1993)

Like Beauchamp and Rife before him, Gaston Naessens (a French microbiologist) states unequivocally, "Germs are not the cause of, but the result of, disease."

—Steven R. Elswick
(*The Amazing Wonders of Gaston Naessens*)

Acceptance of the theory of contagion is contingent upon the germ theory of disease—Nevertheless, the germ theory and the belief of contagion is difficult to overcome since almost everyone's mind has similarly been "infected" by exploitive "health care" industries that have a vested interest in disease and suffering and in perpetuating such erroneous beliefs. Basically the populace believes what the medical establishment wants it to. These false theories maintain demand for drugs, medical and hospital practices and they are the only ones that teach that health is recovered by administrating poisonous drugs. If germs play any role in the causation of disease, it is never a primary one but is always secondary to those causes that lower our resistance or impair health.

—A. Baker, M.A.

My third conclusion is that disease can be cured through the proper use of correct foods. This statement may sound deceptively simple, but I have arrived at it only after intensive study of a highly complex subject: colloid and endocrine chemistry. My conclusions are based on experimental and observational results, gathered through years of successfully treating patients. Occasionally I have resorted to the use of drugs in emergency situations, but those times have been rare. Instead, I have sought to prescribe for my patients' illnesses antidotes which nature has placed at their disposal.

—Bieler, Henry G., M.D.
(*Food Is Your Best Medicine* 1965)

Diseases are crises of purification, of toxic elimination

—Hippocrates
(founder of modern medicine, born in 460 b.c.)

To believe that sickness results solely from the visitation of some itinerant germ or virus and to accept treatment by some poisonous drug is to be found guilty of the most naive superstition.

—Dr. D. Phillips

I have myself, through Natural Hygiene, over 16 years, treated all forms and hundreds of cases of typhus and typhoid fevers, pneumonia, measles and dysentery, and have not lost a single patient. The same is true of scarlet and other fevers. No medicine whatever was given.

—Russell T. Trall, MD (1860)

These diseases (typhoid and pneumonia) are nothing more nor less than a cleansing process—a struggle of the vital powers to relieve the system of its accumulated impurities. The causes of the diseases are constipating foods, contaminated water, atmospheric miasmas, and whatever clogs up the system or befouls the blood. And the day is not far distant when a physician who shall undertake to aid and assist (suppress) nature in her efforts to expel impurities, by the administration of poisons (drugs, medicines, shots, radiation, etc.) will be regarded as an insane idiot. But now this practice is called medical science.

—R. T. Trall, MD (*The Healing Art or Hygienic vs. Drug Medication* 1862)

have we learned *anything* from history?

Do you know the old saying, "He who does not learn from history is destined to repeat it?"

How sad it is that so many people have suffered and died needlessly from diseases that were preventable. We understand now that diseases such as scurvy, beriberi and pellagra were preventable diseases. As if this weren't tragic enough, it seems we have not learned anything from this needless suffering. We know from history that there are diseases that were treated by ridiculous means; treatment that only added to the suffering of the sick and infirmed. If we had only learned from that suffering and the ill treatment of the diseased, and then used the knowledge and experience in treating modern diseases, at least we could feel that we have advanced. It would be so nice to be able to say, "We've come a long way."

In fact, we can say nothing of the kind. Oh we can say that scurvy, beriberi, pellagra, and other "ancient diseases" have been confined to the history books, but there are now other diseases that have taken their place. Cancer, diabetes, and heart disease are claiming more lives with each passing day. These diseases and others are lifestyle issues that are not solved with drugs. There must be a lifestyle change; a permanent change in the way we are living our day to day lives. The right change can stop and reverse even serious degenerative diseases. However, you are the one who has to do it. Consider this: if you suffer with cancer, diabetes, heart disease, high blood pressure, obesity, etc., *you* have the power to change that suffering. As Phillip Day says, "You have to walk the walk."

Three of the degenerative diseases I just mentioned, cancer, heart disease, and diabetes, are the three "big ones," but there are many more that are plaguing thousands. Most diseases, even today, are metabolic dysfunctions of the body.

Phillip Day explains in his teaching, *Cancer, the Winnable War,* that a metabolic dysfunction of the body means that it is a disease that is "wedded to our utilization of food." Scurvy, beriberi, and pellagra are diseases that are metabolic dysfunctions of the body. Each of these diseases were brought on by severe vitamin deficiencies. We have no problem when someone says that scurvy is just a vitamin C deficiency; that pellagra is a lack of niacin; and that beriberi a lack of thiamin. There was a time, though, when there were a handful of people who knew that truth and couldn't get the authorities to listen long enough to believe. There was (and still is) a prejudice against nutritional therapy. During these sad times in our history, authorities refused to believe that nutrition could possibly be the answer to the plagues of diseases that caused so many deaths. These authorities ignored critical information that could have saved many, many lives.

We are appalled to think thousands and thousands of people suffered and died while the knowledge was there *for years* before action was finally taken. It is even more shocking when we understand how some of the treat-

scurvy

ments they used to "help" those suffering were actually worse than the disease itself.

Scurvy is one of the oldest nutritional deficiency diseases known to man. It is a disease that is now known to be an ascorbic acid (vitamin C) deficiency. Vitamin C is essential in the formation of collagen. The symptoms of scurvy all point to what is going on in the body because of the deficiency. There is joint pain, loss of teeth, the mucous membranes bleed, old wounds that have healed can open back up, and former fractures even come apart. Essentially, the connecting tissues of the body pull apart.

When scurvy plagued civilizations such as Egypt, Greece, and Rome, no one suspected that this awful disease was caused by a diet poor in vital nutrients.

Between 1556 and 1857, more than 100 scurvy epidemics spread through Europe. Scurvy was the scourge of sea explorers between the sixteenth and eighteenth centuries, and because rations during military campaigns and long ocean voyages very seldom had adequate amounts of foods containing vitamin C, armies and navies were absolutely devastated, sometimes by as much as 50 percent.

One of the first clues to treating scurvy happened during Jacques Cartier's arrival in Newfoundland in 1536. Many of his men were dying from this epidemic. The native Indians there advised Cartier to give them a potion made from spruce needles. This foliage, which is rich in vitamin C, healed most of the crew.

History tells of different indications that linked

scurvy with diet. Sadly, this knowledge had to be "rediscovered" many, many times until the nineteenth century. In 1742, James Lind, the British naval commander, described miracle cures he encountered with the use of lemon juice. He begged the British navy to institute a program for making citrus foods available on voyages. He was all but ignored.

Many years later, the British navy did adopt Lind's suggested procedure when Captain Cook succeeded in avoiding scurvy completely by giving his sailors lime juice on three voyages between 1768 and 1779. This was such an amazing thing that Captain Cook was presented with the Copley Medal of the Royal Society for his success in bringing back as many sailors from his voyages as had departed. Still, no one knew why citrus juice had such an amazing effect.

The story of scurvy seems to drag on. Account after account is recorded of ships losing most of their crew to this disease, even hundreds of years after others *knew* what needed to be supplied on board to insure protection from scurvy. Armies fared no better. In the late sixteenth century and into the eighteenth century, epidemics of scurvy broke out among Prussian armies, Russians at war between Russians and the Turks, English troops at Quebec, and French soldiers trying to cross the Alps. The common thread in *all* scurvy epidemics was the lack of access to fresh fruits and vegetables.

One particular account of scurvy told about a sailor whose legs were so swollen that the man could not walk. His captain put the man off the ship onto an island, hoping to stop the dreaded scurvy "infection." The captain felt that the poor man was bound to die anyway, but thought that just maybe the rest of the crew would be saved.

The deserted man chewed on fresh grass that he found here and there on the island. A few days later, to his astonishment, he found he could walk a bit! His strength soon returned, eventually he was picked up by a passing ship, and he returned to his home in London. Can you imagine how shocked his former shipmates were when they saw him?!

So, do you think the medical world of those days rejoiced when some people began to put two and two together? No, instead of rejoicing, the medical authorities ridiculed and scorned the idea that scurvy could be prevented by a diet high in vitamin C. They were even able to point to the fact that "the crews of some ships drank lemon juice and still got scurvy." Unfortunately, this was true, but the sailors aboard those ships had boiled the lemon juice, destroying the vitamin C in the juice!

When I was studying about scurvy, I think one of the saddest statements I read was, "Left untreated, scurvy eventually leads to death; fortunately it is extremely easy to address." Wow—*extremely easy* to address. For literally hundreds of years, authorities would not listen to what others had already discovered about the disease; and all because of prejudice against nutritional therapy. It just couldn't be that simple—could it?

beriberi

Another ancient disease caused by poor nutrition is beriberi. Beriberi is a disease involving the nervous system and is caused by a thiamine (vitamin B1) deficiency. Thiamine occurs naturally in unrefined cereals and fresh foods, particularly whole grains, green vegetables and fruit. Symptoms of this severe deficiency include extreme lethargy, fatigue, weight loss, impaired sensory perception, weakness and pain in the limbs, and periods of irregular heart rate. The disease eventually leads to heart failure and death. The word beriberi actually means, "I cannot, I cannot," the word doubled for emphasis. The word itself lets you see how very weak and helpless a person with beriberi must have felt.

Beriberi was found in people whose diet was mostly polished white rice, which is very low in thiamine because the thiamine-bearing husk has been removed. The disease was often found in Asian countries in the nineteenth century and before. Those countries relied heavily on white rice as a staple food.

In Japan, beriberi was named *kakke*. There they thought it resulted from edema of the spinal cord. The Japanese doctor would treat it with acupuncture, applying needles in the calf, and with a poultice-like treatment applied to the back along the line of the spine. The poultice was stuck to a chosen part of the body and then lit to set it smoldering. They believed that it would draw out toxic gases from the body. As the poultice burned down, it raised a blister, which sometimes became infected. This treatment in many cases was worse than the disease itself. Some western doctors included this practice when treating beriberi in colonial territories.

During the time when Pasteur's germ theory was gaining popularity, the Dutch East India Company assigned a team to find the "offending beriberi germ."

They put blood, saliva, and urine under the microscope. They tried everything but found nothing. Finally after nine months, they gave up and went home, leaving their youngest member in charge.

The young man's name was Christian Eijkman. For ten years, he continued to work on the problem. At one point, the chickens where he was stationed came down with what looked like beriberi. They were sick for several months, and some died. Eventually, the rest recovered.

At first, Eijkman did not think much about it. Then something clicked! The chickens got sick after a usual shipment of brown rice did not show up. The cook provided white rice for them. After time went by, the superintendent found out and said "Stop this! White rice is too expensive!" They then switched the chickens back to brown rice—that was about the time the surviving chickens recovered.

Polished white rice was a nineteenth century refinement. Eijkman began to think maybe that held the secret. He went to local jails to check menus. Where they served brown rice, there was little beriberi. Where they had only white rice, beriberi was rampant. After testing his theory, Eijkman soon established that those people who ate the unrefined brown rice did not get beriberi while those who ate the supposedly better, polished rice did.

Eijkman was not the first person to attempt to convince others that beriberi was a nutritional problem. There were others years before who saw the relationship between the disease and what made up a person's diet. As in the case of scurvy, there would be much more suffering and death before authorities would finally listen.

Again, just as in the story of scurvy, this nutritional

explanation seemed too simple to believe and was rejected. Eijkman did not give up and doggedly supported his claims with more research. It's funny, though; he thought the difference in the two kinds of rice was that the white rice must hold some kind of poison, and the brown-colored bran must carry the antidote! He solved the immediate problem, but his reasoning was way off the mark.

It wasn't until several years later that a Pole named Casimir Funk understood what was happening. The husks contained a nutrient (thiamin) that our bodies must have but cannot produce on its own. He found that these nutrients come in other foods as well. Funk is credited in giving nutrients the name "vitamins."

pellagra

Most people do not even know what pellagra is, it is so far removed from our times. Pellagra is Italian for "rough skin." Sadly, this malady brought much more than just rough skin for its victims. It eventually led to insanity and death.

We now know that pellagra is caused by a lack of niacin, or vitamin B_3, in the diet. Niacin is found in green leafy vegetables, nuts, seeds, and other foods. Pellagra was found largely in populations who relied on the extensive use of corn for food.

More importantly than this was the character of the meal ground from the corn. Before 1900 most of the meal was locally ground in grist meals that were usually water driven. Water-ground meal was coarsely ground, and much of the germ and hull of the grain were retained in the meal. About the turn of the century, cornmeal was finely ground by large milling companies. This "western meal" was thoroughly de-germinated to keep it from becoming rancid during storage and shipment. The meal looked better, kept better, and made more palatable bread; unfortunately, this processing also destroyed all of the corn's vital nutrients.

Pellagra begins with weakness, skin rash, mouth sores, and a loss of appetite. However, it gradually worsens with a severe inflammation of the skin, mental confusion, and diarrhea. Left unchecked, death follows.

In the beginning of this terrible disease, most scientists believed it to be caused by toxins, possibly in wet or spoiled maize. They spent many wasted years searching for this elusive germ. We are seeing a pattern with the germ theory aren't we? People down through history have been so ready to attribute diseases to the germ theory. Time after time, though, it is disproved; yet, somehow the theory never dies the death it deserves.

Pellagra victims were shunned as "lepers." The pellagra epidemic had created a "pellagra phobia." The diagnosis of pellagra usually resulted in social isolation of the patient, with the patient falling into complete despair. Some hospitals even refused admission to pellagra victims. Tennessee hospitals were the first to isolate them as patients. Other states soon followed suit. The unsuspecting patient was given a plethora of unpleasant and illogical therapeutic options. Arsenic, strychnine, quinine, partial appendectomy, and static electric shock were some of the things prescribed for the pellagra patient.

Pellagra had always been a problem in the American south where corn and cornmeal were staples in the diet. It was not until 1907, though, when a major epidemic broke out that the government launched serious investigative studies. Joseph Goldberger was a doctor who in 1913 devoted himself to finding a solution to this terrible scourge.

Again, it was Casimir Funk who had already suggested that pellagra might be caused by a poor diet, and Dr. Goldberger and his associates agreed. They found pellagra attacked people who mainly, because of poverty, had diets that consisted of cornmeal, salt pork, lard, and molasses.

Goldberger conducted experiments with different groups of people. He modified diets in institutions to show he could induce and reverse pellagra by diet alone.

Around 1914, it was commonly thought that pellagra was an infectious and communicable disease. When Goldberger first went to the Deep South and saw the victims there, he was shocked at their condition. Even though the surroundings were filthy and flies were swarming everywhere, still he did not feel this was the cause of the disease, and he was not biased by the preexisting opinions. He still believed it was a dietary problem. He found that in the mental institutions many of the patients had pellagra while the staff did not. The staff and the patients had close contact, but the staff stayed relatively free of the disease. Upon further investigation, he found that the diet of the staff was varied and much better than the diet of the patients, who lived mostly on cereal grains.

Newspapers in the area even reported Goldberger's findings. Shocking, but not terribly surprising in light of the pattern we are beginning to see, some government studies actually recorded that pellagra was probably caused by the bite of a fly. Goldberger was frustrated by this, but he determined to prove his findings in any way he could. He knew unless he could somehow convince authorities that pellagra was indeed a dietary problem, thousands of people would continue to die.

To show to his critics once and for all that pellagra was not communicable, Goldberger exposed sixteen volunteers, including his wife, to blood, urine, feces, and epidermal scales of pellagrous lesions. Pellagra did not develop in *any* of the volunteers. Finally, people were convinced germs were not the culprit, but it was poor diet that held the answer to pellagra. Joseph Goldberger stripped pellagra of its mystery and its myths. He discovered and was able to prove the true cause of pellagra. He stepped on quite a number of medical toes when his research experiments showed that diet and not germs caused the disease.

Scurvy, pellagra, and beriberi no longer plague our nation as they once did. Many years were wasted and thousands of lives lost needlessly while the authorities of that time were being convinced that something as simple as diet could truly be the answer. It's sad to say, but it seems that it might have been an insult to pride and intelligence to have to admit they had missed something so glaringly obvious.

The past is history that is true. The past cannot be changed; but when we ignore and fail to respect the past, we put the future at risk. Even though the past cannot be changed, it is still valuable for what it can teach us. Learning from the past can be a cornerstone of wisdom. Repeating the mistakes of the past because of stubborn pride and even worse, greed, is unforgivable.

Do you ever ponder what history books will say about how we treated our patients; patients diagnosed with cancer and heart disease; patients living and dying with diabetes? What kind of review will they give to the treatments we had for these patients? Can you imagine what future generations will think of the way we poisoned, burned, and cut up cancer patients? Do you wonder? I do. I wonder and I grieve. I grieve the thousands upon thousands of people who have suffered and died needlessly of a mysterious disease; a disease that wasn't so mysterious after all.

the choice of health care

The last chapter told some of the history of diseases in our nation. In writing about the mess we have in our county with health and disease, we have seen how people are depending on medical doctors and pharmaceutical drugs for the answers to disease. We are going down the same road that led to so many unnecessary deaths in our past. After so much sadness and despair, quite frankly I was ready to move on to talking about a happier subject; which is how to live out our lives in great health.

For some reason, I found I could not go on to that subject until I address this topic that is so disturbing yet probably not something most parents have even thought about. This chapter is about the choice we have, or more correctly, don't have regarding the health care of our children.

We are now reading in our newspaper headlines and hearing in news reports about forced medical care on children in our nation. A few years ago, I would hear a report here and there about an underage child being forced, against the parents' wishes, to receive traditional medical care. Those were always stories I just happened to hear.

One story was on a conservative talk radio show. The host of the show had a young man as his guest who was being taken to court by child protective services to force him to receive chemotherapy that he had determined he did not want to receive. This young man was sixteen years old, and because he was not of legal age, the courts were saying he did not have the right to choose his own medical care. They were saying he must do what his doctor said was right for him. This young man had already been through rounds of chemotherapy, and still his cancer had returned. He had decided that he did not want to go the chemotherapy route again. He had already experienced the horrors of that and wanted to avoid living through that again. He knew the chemotherapy was not truly curing the cancer. He desired to try nutritional therapy for the cancer that had returned in his body.

I remember the host of the show was completely shocked. He said, "Now you are telling me that if you lose this battle with the courts, they will come and basically arrest you and force you to take chemotherapy; they will strap you down and force the medicine into your veins. Is that what you are telling me?" The boy sadly told the host yes; that is exactly what would happen to him if he lost the battle.

I read another story about forced medical care in our local newspaper. A father brought his daughter to our city to have alternative treatment for a cancer she had. He saw what radiation was doing to her body and he wanted something better for her. He wanted to stop the burning and poisoning of her body. The authorities were trying to have him arrested and his daughter put into foster care so she "could receive the treatment she needed," the treatment the *medical authorities* said she needed.

In 1998, a little two-year-old boy was diagnosed with a brain tumor. After he endured two brain surgeries, his parents sought the best therapy for him. They found a non-toxic therapy that had been proven successful in treating pediatric brain cancer. The FDA, however, denied them access to this treatment. It seems the oncologist had already determined that without the latest and greatest chemotherapy treatment, this little boy's cancer would return. The parents did not want this toxic treatment for their son, but they had no choice. When they hesitated to bring their son in for chemo, the oncologists began gearing up to take the baby away from them by a court order. The little boy went through three months of chemotherapy and died a month later. The parents learned later that the exact chemo protocol the oncologists had given their son had been *proven* to be ineffective in pediatric brain tumors many years before.

The stories of forced medical treatment are becoming more blatant. The media and many people are siding with the government in saying that parents are being negligent if they do not care for their child in the way the doctor has decided is best. It seems we are supposed to turn over our parental rights, the right to care for our children—the children God has entrusted to *us*, to the government.

More recently, the headlines tell of a thirteen-year-old boy who is defying authorities in the choice of treatment of his cancer diagnosis. The mother of the boy is being vilified and accused of "neglecting" her son because she wants to use nutritional therapy to heal her son's cancer instead of the chemotherapy she saw was poisoning his body. The boy took one round of chemotherapy and decided for himself that he would not take any more. The courts have decided that the boy is too young to decide for himself. The judge ruled in favor of the doctor in charge of the boy's medical care. The doctor has said chemotherapy is the boy's only chance of beating the disease.

It seems we, as parents, no longer have the choice in how we will care for our children if and when they are sick. If we take them to a medical doctor and then question or disagree with the doctor regarding medical treatment for them, they can be taken away from us, put into a foster home, and we can be arrested for endangering the health and welfare of our children.

I think of a lady who once said to me, "I am not afraid of cancer anymore. After seeing the success you had with nutritional treatment, I know what I would do if I ever got cancer." This lady made it clear she did not want to change the way she ate until she *had* to. At the time I just thought, "Well that is her choice. If she ever does *have* to change her lifestyle because of a diagnosis, I hope there is time to turn it around, but ultimately, it really is her choice."

Lately, in light of all that is going on with the control of our children, I have thought more about that discussion I had with her. This lady has small children, and she is not only making the choice for herself, but for her children. She is taking a chance with their health. While it is true, for now at least, if she is ill and goes to the doctor, this lady will have the choice whether to receive traditional medical treatment or not; she most likely will not have that choice with her children's care. If her children become ill and are diagnosed by a medical doctor, she will have to allow that doctor to treat her children with the treatment *the doctor* chooses, or risk being labeled a criminal. The doctor can use his authority to have the children taken away and put into state run foster care.

For more reasons than just living a long life and having great energy and vitality, we must act in a responsible way, if only for the sake of our children. Be responsible for not just your health, but for the health of those God has entrusted to you. Learn the Master's design for our bodies. Teach your children how to eat healthy and why it is important. Live and pursue a life that will be pleasing to the One who created life … and enjoy a lifetime of no regrets.

who really wants great health?

When I see yet another plea for donations to help with a cure for diabetes, cancer, heart disease, etc., I feel so saddened. So many people are looking, searching for a cure for themselves or for a loved one, but very few understand that we ourselves are responsible for our own health.

We look to scientists and researchers to find this elusive "cure" while we keep going about our business doing what we've been doing all of our lives; we are creating the diseases our bodies have to endure. I want to dance and shout "Listen, look—the 'cure' is here!" It is so incredibly simple it would almost seem unbelievable. In fact, it is unbelievable to most of us.

The fact is, it is true that we have everything we need to have the abounding health so many are craving yet not achieving. It is an exciting yet sobering thought.

One morning, I received an e-mail asking for a donation to help in the search for a cure. This time it was for diabetes. The man who sent it also sent a picture of himself. He was in a wheelchair and probably weighed over 500 pounds. I happen to know a little something about this man. He is so heavy he cannot move from his wheelchair to his bed without help. He cannot go to the bathroom without help.

I just cannot imagine living life that way. The daily

choices he is making are keeping him in that wheelchair and making him depend on others to physically move him from bed to wheelchair then back to bed again. If that were not enough to make my heart grieve, this e-mail making a plea for donations for a cure for his diabetes does! Who does not know that diabetes is a direct result of the way a person eats? My first reaction was, "It is pretty bold to eat however you want and then ask people to send money to find a 'cure' for your disease."

As these kinds of thoughts went through my head, I suddenly realized, "This man does not know or understand that it is the food he is eating, the way he is living his life that is causing the life he has to live. He is imprisoned by a culture and society that has taught us for generations that it doesn't matter what we eat. Our world tells us that we should satisfy our taste buds however we like and that we should be able to eat whenever and whatever we want. We are told illness and diseases come upon us as we age, or we get sick because of environmental toxins, or red dye number whatever! We are never taught that we are choosing the future we will live with each bite we put into our mouths.

It would seem too that we'd rather not hear how important nutrition is. We'd rather believe it doesn't matter too much what we eat. I love how Norman Walker put it in his book, *Diet and Salad,* "Human nature is all too often obstinate and stubborn, refusing to be confused by facts, and is traditionally oblivious or heedless to experience, and to good judgment."

When I think about how much I'd love to help people with health, I realize that first they have to be motivated. Then they have to be educated. I believe many people would begin to make good choices concerning food if they truly understood that they can make a difference in their health. So often, though, even when someone does get motivated to do something, they are overwhelmed and do not know *what* to do. It can be confusing to try to understand how to begin eating healthy.

There are many differing opinions as to what healthy eating looks like. It is not enough to look around and find some diet we think we can live with that sounds healthy. We must begin to understand what real food is and how it nourishes and rebuilds the body. It is equally important to understand what junk food is and how it tears down and sickens the body. To understand both is the beginning of a change. It can be the beginning of abounding health; the beginning of abundant health for life!

The only people I know who truly have been completely healed of disease and are living their lives with abundant health are the ones who have taken responsibility for their health. They woke up and realized that traditional medical doctors do not have the answers for health. They only have the "answers" for disease. They can teach you how to live with a disease. Who wants to do that? Who wants to live the life we have in doctors' offices waiting to be scanned, tested, and prodded? I think it is pretty safe to say that no one wants to live that way.

Traditional doctors give out prescriptions for chemicals to help us live with a disease. Then in the case of cancer, we are living the rest of our lives waiting for cancer to come back or spread. We are waiting for the cancer to get to the point where they can no longer treat it. Then we die.

It's the same thing with diabetes. We are taught to treat the disease and live with it until we get to the point where it cannot be treated anymore and we die. I do not want to be taught to live with a disease. I want to overcome that disease and live in health! I truly believe that is what most people want…if they only knew it was possible. The great news is it is not only possible, but it is the way God intended for us to live out our lives.

When I was diagnosed with cancer, I think one of the things that frightened me the most was that I believed I would be living the rest of my life going through scans and tests to watch for the cancer's return. Even if I totally beat the disease through traditional medicine's answers of surgery, chemotherapy, and radiation (traditional medicine's only answers for cancer), I'd still be living my life in cancer's shadow.

When I discovered the real answer for cancer, I was so excited; and the excitement stemmed from the fact that I did not have to live my life watching for cancer's return. I could totally beat the disease and never look back. This is only true if I would be willing to take responsibility for my own health. I truly believe that is the missing factor here. We must be willing to take responsibility.

As I look at what people are doing to be healed and to live in health, I see many things. I see people looking to doctors, doing fundraising events for "cures," searching the Internet for the latest alternative to traditional medicine, attending healing services, etc. I know the last one may seem out of place because I do believe in God's healing. I believe in His miracles. What I do not believe in is asking Him to heal us but being unwilling to do our part. I think about that and I get excited when I realize that most people want to do their part, if they only knew what to do.

While I see people taking all these different measures to attain health, what I don't see are very many people who know and understand that they can regain their health through proper nourishment of the body. Most people will admit they do not eat right, but those same people do not fully understand what the food they are eating is doing to their body, and they have no idea what food they should eat to bring life to the body; food that will allow their body to be the amazing self-healing body our Creator made it to be.

I know eating can be a fun part of family celebrations, and to a point, that's okay; but eating has become an obsession. We are literally eating ourselves to death.

It would be one thing if we just ate ourselves to death. What is happening, though, is we are eating ourselves to ill health, disease, and then death. There are years in between where we are suffering and living a pitiful life.

Can you imagine what it would be like if we suddenly realized that we can make a dramatic difference in the state of our health with just changing that one part of our lives—namely, the way we eat? We probably would not recognize ourselves! When we think how much of our lives in this country revolves around food, it is eye opening.

So much of our economy is based on food. We have restaurants of all kinds on every corner. Grocery stores are packed to overflowing with more junk food than real food. Gas stations are no longer just gas stations. They need to have an abundance of junk food to please those of us who don't just come in to buy gas for our cars. Almost any store you go in has a certain amount of junk food available for us to be able to satisfy our eating urges.

Then there's the industry that thrives on the illness and disease people cause to their bodies by eating, eating, eating. On Phillip Day's CD he states, "The cancer industry is making over a billion dollars a year just treating and researching cures for that disease."

What would happen if more of us would suddenly discover that the cure is in our own hands and if we toughened up and took charge of our own health? It is a very exciting thought! The rich life that is there for us is exciting, even though it may seem out of reach. However, it is only out of reach because we do not know how or what to change.

When I think of how God must feel when He sees us struggling with health issues the way we do, I imagine how sad He must feel. He created us to be in health. He gave us all the answers right in His Word. The knowledge of how to live our lives in wonderful health is all right there. But we must take the responsibility. We must decide that we would rather be strong and bold when it comes to living the life He has for us, than sickly and defeated. God's Word says, "My people are destroyed for lack of knowledge" (Hosea 4:6 KJV).

People as a whole do not know and fully understand the role nutrition and healthy habits play in living our life abundantly. We have lived our lives for so long letting doctors, the medical establishment, and government studies tell us what we need to do about diseases and even what we should and should not be eating. We go the medical route for our health because that is familiar…that seems less overwhelming. How much do we *really* know about traditional medicine? What we do not know can indeed hurt us.

What most of us do not realize is that doctors are trained by the very pharmaceutical companies that make money from all the medications prescribed. Doctors are trained to treat diseases and to treat them with what the pharmaceutical companies provide. In a first-year pharmacology class at Harvard Medical School, one student in particular grew very frustrated as the professor promoted the benefits of cholesterol drugs and would belittle students who asked about the side effects. This student later discovered something very interesting about this professor by searching online. This professor was not only a full-time member of the Harvard Medical faculty, but he was also a paid consultant to ten drug companies, *including* five makers of the very cholesterol drugs he liked to talk about in his teachings.

More recently, a ranking Republican senator who was on the Senate finance committee was looking into financial ties between the pharmaceutical industry and the academic physicians who, for the most part, determine the market value of prescription drugs. He didn't have to look very hard. He found information about a doctor who was the professor of psychiatry at a prominent medical school *and* chief of pediatric psychopharmacology at a large hospital. Thanks to this doctor, children as young as two years old are now being diagnosed with bipolar disorder and treated with a cocktail of powerful drugs. Many of these drugs are not even approved by the FDA for that purpose, and *none* of them are approved for children below ten years old.

There are accounts after accounts of the ties between pharmaceutical companies and doctors, and just as importantly, these same pharmaceutical companies and the training of doctors.

The story is much the same with studies that show we need certain food groups to be healthy. Government studies are funded by special interest groups. Who decided that dairy should be a food group? Who influences those studies to say that we need a certain amount of animal protein? The only studies that are worth our attention are the ones that are funded by private individuals with no group profiting from their findings.

Much like the senator found when he went looking, the facts are not hard to find when you really want to know. For the most part, we just do not take the time to find out who is doing these studies and who is behind the information we are getting from our doctors. We are ignorantly following the findings and the advice; sometimes to our *death*. That sounds very dramatic, but it is true more often than we'd like to think. We are like the naïve children following the pied piper. If it sounds good, and even sometimes when it doesn't sound so good, we'll try it; especially if it doesn't involve too much changing of the way we eat!

This is even true with studies being done with alternative health measures. We are willing to buy in to alternative measures, maybe in part because we do not have to really change the way we live. We can just buy this new vitamin drink, take a handful of special supplements, or have some treatment, and still be able to consume all the food we love to eat! Do these things get us to the point where we are living abundantly? No, and the reason is we have not taken responsibility. We have listened to what others say we need to do, and we do it.

Again, one reason we are so willing to do it is because it does not truly involve changing our lifestyle and taking full responsibility for our health. In the alternative health field, much like traditional medicine, we are willing to pay someone else to tell us what to take, what new supplement we need to buy to have health.

We are still willing to live in poor health, even to the point of being in a wheelchair and having to have someone come and get us in and out of bed. I say that unwillingness to change is only one reason we let someone else tell us what we need to do in the area of our health because I feel that most of us would be willing to do something different if we just knew what to do.

We need to believe that we can live out our whole life with great health and energy. We have believed the lie that as we get older we can count on living with a lack of vitality, in ill health, and even in the state of disease. We are no longer surprised when people are diagnosed with a grave disease. We almost expect it. Oh, we are still looking to doctors and researchers to come up with the reasons and cures for diseases, but we are not actively seeking it ourselves.

Could it be possible that if we discovered the truth, we'd be accountable to make some changes? What if we found out the truth, kept eating the typical diet of mostly cooked and junk food, and then continued on down the road to doctors, medicines, even to the point of asking for donations to fund research for a cure? Wouldn't that be living a lie? Do the foods we are eating really taste so wonderful that we are willing to sacrifice a life of health and energy for them? With knowledge comes responsibility. We would not be able to live with ourselves if we knew the truth of what the food we eat is doing to our body and still did not change directions.

If we could see right away how eating that junk food is affecting our immediate health, then we probably would steer clear of it. If we felt the effect immediately when we eat those chips, that cheeseburger, those fries, etc. then we would probably feel very motivated to never eat those foods again.

Part of the problem is some of those foods give us good feelings right away. Feelings of comfort and pleasure (and lethargy!) do accompany the eating of these kinds of foods; and since we are not in great health anyway, we do not know what great health feels like. We have nothing to compare to those feelings of comfort and even lethargy. If we could get a clear picture of what those choices are doing to our bodies and then see how we *could be* living our lives, I think then we would have the courage to make those changes once and for all!

The fact is, we are not thinking about the long run. The future looks pretty bleak right now for growing older. While we may be living longer in the terms of years, there's really not much vitality to those years. We see many Americans over the age of 40 living their lives managing one or more chronic illnesses and on several prescription medications. Do we really want to look forward to living out our lives the way the majority of Americans do as they age? Wouldn't it be so much better to be excited about growing older, knowing we can have great health and energy at any age? Do we just expect our energy and strength to decrease as we age? Are we expecting to have ill health and disease at some point in our lives?

We can look forward to an exciting life of great health and energy if we will educate ourselves and then take responsibility and make these changes. Once the changes are made and we determine to do the right thing no matter what our taste buds are saying, then those taste buds actually change and we begin to want the very things that our bodies need. We actually begin to crave the good things that God made for us in the beginning; we will crave the food He created to fuel our bodies to allow us live our lives to truly honor Him.

Isn't that what we were created to do anyway? We are supposed to be living our lives in a way that will bring glory to Him. How do we do that while struggling with poor health? Let's make the determination to live our lives to honor Him. Let's start with making wise choices about our lifestyle, even though it will mean completely changing the way we think about food!

what is great health?

Now that we have determined we must take responsibility for our own health, we need to ask the question "What is health?" Is health just the absence of disease? I hear people say, "My health is great," and at the same time they are bone tired after a normal day's activities, or they battle colds and the flu, have problems with weight gain, are easily depressed or emotional, etc.

At the other end of the spectrum there are people who are astonished when they are diagnosed with cancer, diabetes, heart problems, or some other chronic disease because they "haven't been sick a day in their lives." These people don't get the typical colds and the flu like others do all around them, so they assume they are in good health.

One afternoon, I was in the ladies' dressing room in a department store. In the room next to mine I could clearly hear a woman in distress. The manager of the department had called for help saying that there was a lady having difficulty breathing. I went over and prayed with the lady and held her hand until help came. During this time, the manager was on the phone with EMS asking the lady questions and relaying the answers. At one point the manager asked the lady, "Are you in good health?" The lady answered, "I'm extremely healthy!"

I was shocked!

First of all, how could you answer "I'm extremely healthy," when it's obvious to all those around that you are having a heart attack? My next thought was, "How very sad. Here is another person deceived into thinking they are in good health just because they have not been diagnosed with an illness or disease."

We need to change our thinking of what it means to live our lives in great health. Being healthy does not just mean the absence of disease. We can evaluate our health somewhat by the way we feel. Are we tired way too often? Do we have many aches and pains? Do we have strength and energy throughout the day? The answers to these questions will give us clues to how healthy we really are.

Even our emotional state reveals our health. Are we truly joyful about each new day? Do we feel excitement when thinking about our future? The health of our body will dictate how much emotional energy we have. When the body is struggling, even in areas we don't know about, we don't have the emotional energy we need to be joyful and excited. Do you ever feel depressed and you just don't know why? It could be lack of health in the body.

As I briefly mentioned above, many people believe they are in great health because they are the ones in their family who never get colds, the flu, viruses, etc. We need to fully understand the fallacy of this thinking. When I was diagnosed with cancer, I was in shock. I know anyone who is diagnosed with such a grave disease would be in shock for a time, but it was more than just the severity of the diagnosis that shocked me. I was the one in my family who never got sick. There was one winter when literally everyone in my family had the flu, except for me. I remember thinking, "I guess I am the healthy one!"

abounding health naturally

Gradually, though, I began to understand that just because we never get colds and other minor illnesses it does not mean we are in great health. In fact, that very thing can signal something major going on in the body. The body can be in such distress in dealing with a major issue that it does not have the energy to have a cold.

Yes, having a cold takes energy. The body has to have the energy to spare to have a cold. If the body is tied up with major things like cancer or heart disease, it is doing all it can to just stay alive; it cannot expend any energy for a cold. We all know that the diagnosis of cancer is not the beginning of cancer. Cancer had its start way before we knew about it. The body certainly knew about it, though, and was doing its best with what it had to deal with it.

Let's not be complacent, though, and think because we have lots of colds that we are healthy! No, someone who has one cold after another, infections, viruses, and other minor ailments is certainly not healthy. Nor does this mean that the body is not also dealing with a chronic disease like cancer. I do not want to lead people to believe that because they have many colds a year that "at least my body must not have cancer." We just never know how much cleansing energy the individual body has.

We must wake up to what health truly is and is not on both ends. Let's not live in blindness and ignorance. I can remember years ago thinking, "If I have cancer, I just don't want to know about it!" What a crazy thought! The sooner we know about a disease like that, the better chance our body will have enough energy to fight it and gain health again. Even better, why not do something about our health now, before we find out something is terribly wrong?

I am not saying there are any promises of living to be a hundred. I know that just because we nourish our bodies with all the right foods, get plenty of fresh air and sunshine, exercise daily, have a great attitude, etc. does not guarantee that God will give us a long life. Of course, God can take us home any time He wants.

What I *am* saying is I want to live my life, until the moment I die, in great health. Deuteronomy 34:7 says, "And Moses was an hundred and twenty years old when he died: his eye was not dim, nor his natural force abated." God made these bodies to last a lifetime. It is not right to have our bodies wear out years before we die. We have grown accustomed to thinking that as we get older our bodies start to break down. This may be a common thing, but it is certainly not natural. It is not God's plan for us to live much of our life battling sickness and disease.

Our body is not a machine. It is a creation of God. Our body is comprised of living cells that were designed by God to be nourished with living food. In Genesis 1:29, our Creator plainly shows us His plan to nourish our body. "And God said, Behold I have given you every herb bearing seed, which is upon the face of all the earth, and every tree, in which is the fruit of a tree yielding seed; to you it shall be for food."

Psalm 139:14 says, "I will praise thee; for I am fearfully and wonderfully made: marvelous are thy works and that my soul knows right well." God made our bodies "fearfully and wonderfully"! How exciting it is to be able to live our lives with no worries about failing health.

Oh yes, our future is in God's hands, but when we obey Him, and live our lives making healthy choices, we can live in joy and fully expect great health. God has given us the gift of health.

We earn the disease we create in our bodies by the poor choices we make. We earn disease through either ignorance or apathy. Many people just do not know what good nutrition is. Many more people just really do not care.

My desire is to help people replace the ignorance with knowledge of how to eat properly for great health. It will be your job to get rid of the apathy. It is our choice.

We need to remember this, though, when we call out to our heavenly Father for healing; as we cry out to Him, are we also asking Him what our responsibility is in our health? Are we willing to obey when He shows us our responsibility?

why we should eat for great health

We have determined we do want to be in great health. We now understand better what great health really is. So how do we need to be eating for great health? Before we get deeply in to what we need to be eating, I'd like to explain the why. It is important to know what is going on in our body when we eat poorly, so we have the motivation to be consistent with eating correctly.

Especially in the beginning of all the change, it can be difficult to stick with the things we know are good for us. Later on it gets easier because, as I mentioned earlier, the taste buds will change and pretty soon the things that are good for us are the things we begin to crave. Don't you wonder why it is that some people just really hate the taste of fresh fruits and vegetables? If this is the food that is the best fuel for our bodies, why is it, then, some people just can't stand the taste?

It is a very simple explanation. It is because as the body gets more toxic and clogged with all the junk we feed it, the taste buds also get toxic and clogged. Our taste buds are not tasting the junk food we feed it for what it really is … junk! That is why it is so hard for people to stay the course when they go on a diet. The taste buds do not ever get cleaned out enough to let us enjoy the good food we know we need to eat.

Also, why is it there are those people who have allergies to some fruits and vegetables? How could someone be allergic to the very foods created to be fuel for our bodies?

One possible explanation for this is cleansing. When you give the body food in its raw form, you are supplying your body with amazing energy. This food not only has its own enzymes available to digest, but it has live nutrients. When you give live nutrients to a body that is not used to having such wonderful nutrition, the body is going to do some work. The more cleansing that needs to be done and the more live nutrition you give your body, the more work it can do!

Of course, you cannot just go blindly about eating raw foods and having allergic reactions. This is not good for the body either. Use common sense and eat whatever raw foods you can without too much discomfort. Just know this, though, the body needs to cleanse, and there will be times of discomfort. Keep telling yourself this—the pay-off is well worth it!

Most of us have figured out long ago that ice cream, donuts, cheeseburgers and French fries are not good for us, but we do not really understand why. We all are sure that raw vegetables and fruits are much better for us than pastries, chips, and candy, but do we know why?

Before we get in to why junk food is so bad for our health, I feel that I need to make a clear distinction in the difference in real food and junk food. What is real food? What is junk food? How can we tell the difference?

In Dr. Robbins' audio teaching, *Eating for Health and Wellness*, he says that real food is compatible with the body. In no way does it take away from the body, but

abounding health naturally

contributes to the building up of health and maintaining life. It contains nothing that is harmful, toxic, or non-usable by the body.

Real food is the total package. Real food must meet all of the following qualifications: (1) It must be grown by nature, of the plant kingdom; (2) you must be able to eat it without processing it in any way; and (3) you must be able to eat an entire meal of just that one substance and thoroughly enjoy it. For example, it is not offensive to the taste buds. The taste buds are our primary defense mechanism to keep out toxins. We naturally have a sweet tooth; this is nature's way of attracting us to our naturally right diet. The problem with trusting our taste buds is when the body gets sick and run down our taste buds get sluggish and they cannot tell us what real food is. When someone tells me they do not like the taste of fruit, then I know they must have a very toxic body.

So what is the total package the body needs for great health? Why do we eat the food God created to be fuel for these bodies?

We eat food for glucose, which is the energy, the fuel for our body. We also eat food for protein; protein is for building and repair work. Fatty acids are the next thing we need. Those are the building components of the body tissues. Next we need minerals. These are the catalysts of building components; they help the body work more efficiently. Then there are the enzymes (vitamins); these increase efficiency. Last, we need water. Water is the medium for chemical processes.

Real food must meet all these requirements. Raw fruits and vegetables, nuts, and seeds meet all these criteria. The package is complete; yes, even protein is there in just the right amount for our bodies. God created living foods to be the perfect fuel for our living bodies. Anything less is at best a neutral food and even worse, a junk food.

Junk foods are foods that do not meet all these requirements and do not promote life and health. Junk foods are disease producing because they are missing things the body needs to make use of the food. The body then has to complete the package by borrowing from its own reserves and its own tissue. Junk foods also usually have substances in them that cost the body energy and nutrients in order to be able to eliminate them.

By having to borrow from its own reserves and its own tissue, the body then creates deficiencies. We don't notice this as a problem right away. Over time, it becomes a big problem. When the body gets so run down and depleted of its reserves, ill health and diseases begin.

The substances in junk foods that cost the body greatly in energy and nutrients are called toxins. A toxin is any substance which is foreign to the body that the body cannot use in any way for maintaining life. The body must pull from its own reserves of energy to eliminate them. We pay a big price when we eat food that has toxins, or any food that is not a complete package for that matter. The price we pay is ill health and disease.

So now we know. It is not a matter of just saying this is not good for me or this is bad for me. Now we know that the body must deal with everything we eat and drink. Whether we make wise choices or foolish choices, those choices will determine whether we will live our lives in health or succumb to ill health and disease.

We can see from history that our health in this

country is going downhill. In the early 1900s, 30 percent of the adults age forty and older were being diagnosed with chronic diseases. These are diseases such as cancer, heart disease, and diabetes. Today, with the doctor-to-patient ratio higher than ever, and with more money being spent on medical care than any other country, you'd think things would be looking better, right? In fact, today over 70 percent of adults forty years old and above are being diagnosed with a chronic disease, and in many cases not just one disease, but two. As Dr. Robbins says in his CD set *Nutrition and Its Relation to Health*, "We are now, not surprisingly, in the worst epidemic of chronic disease we have ever known."

Keep in mind that it's not just as we age that our bodies are falling in to bad health. It seems we are hearing about more and more children filling cancer hospitals. Babies are being born with heart disease, diabetes, and even cancer. Why are we seeing our young people dying so suddenly with grave diseases?

In the 1940s, a medical doctor by the name of Francis M. Pottinger financed his own research to determine the effects processed foods have on the body. He took 900 cats and divided them in to five groups. Two of the groups he fed raw food. Three of the groups he fed denatured, processed food. The results he got were simply amazing. With groups one and two, the raw food groups, he saw every generation of cats from the first to the fourth live healthy throughout their lives. With groups three through five, the processed food groups, he saw the first generation of cats develop disease late in life. The second generation of cats developed diseases in the middle of life. The third generation developed diseases at the beginning of life, with many of the cats dying before six months of age. There was no fourth generation of cats. The cats in the third generation were either born sterile or the fourth generation cats were aborted before birth.

This is a startling example of what is happening in our country. As I stated earlier, we are seeing younger and younger friends and family members succumb to illness and disease. While we are distressed when we hear of a child or baby who has cancer, diabetes, or heart disease, we are not particularly shocked anymore. Even more sobering is the fact that we are passing the 25 percent mark of childbearing couples who cannot reproduce. We often hear of someone we know and love who wants to have children and for some reason or another cannot.

I wrote about our trouble with infertility in the first chapter of this book. I also had a couple of cousins who wanted children and were never able to conceive. I remember my mother saying, "This just seems so strange. When I was young, it was very rare that a couple could not have children. We knew of people who wanted children and were not able to have them, but we always thought of them as very different. Now it seems we are hearing more and more of people who cannot have babies. It just seems so strange."

I never thought much about my mom's statement until after I started learning about ill health and disease and why and how it happens. I remember how sad I felt when I compared the health of our country to Dr. Pottinger's cat experiments. Do you wonder what generation we are now experiencing? It is a sobering thought, isn't it?

I often ponder how different my life would be if I had understood the concepts of good health and eating early in my life. Regardless, I can truly say I am grateful for everything I have experienced. Yes, I am even grateful for the period of my life when I was diagnosed with cancer. God took me through a scary, painful time, and through it He taught me many life lessons. Just one of those lessons was why and how to feed this body He created with the food He created especially for it!

what we should eat for great health

I have already talked just a bit about what makes food a "real" food. I'm going to repeat myself just a bit here because I believe I do need to drive this truth home. We must educate ourselves as to what real food is and what it is not before we can talk about what we should be eating for great health.

Remember earlier I gave three points that determined if food is a "real" food. (1) It must be grown by nature, of the plant kingdom; (2) you must be able to eat it without processing it in any way; and (3) you must be able to eat an entire meal of just that one substance and thoroughly enjoy it. Just putting a food through these three test points will eliminate much of what we as Americans are eating on a daily basis. In fact, many people at this point will think to themselves, "What is there to eat, then?" The answer is plenty—and it is all good, just as our Creator said when He created it. He saw what He had made and it was good!

Eat those things that God created to be food for us. Eat them as close to nature as possible, before they were processed and changed into something men (and women) thought might be better.

We always get into trouble when we think we can improve on what God has created. Man has taken things that God created to be food for our bodies and made them more "convenient." I especially fail to see how you could possibly make the beautiful fruits God made in the beginning any more convenient than He did. He gave us such a gift in His creation, and we have polluted and destroyed it. We took live fruits and vegetables, nuts and seeds and processed them in such a way as to destroy all the life in them. To have living bodies, you *must* eat live foods.

When I think of what God created for us to eat, the food He made to fuel our bodies, I think of Genesis 1:29. This scripture says, "And God said, See, I have given you every plant yielding seed that is on the face of all the land and every tree with seed in its fruit; you shall have them for food." God, from the very beginning of creation, had a plan for us; a plan that would allow us to live our lives in health if we would just stay with that plan. There can be no argument that we have drifted far from that original plan of God's best.

After the fall, when sin entered into the scheme of things, vegetation was added to our diet. Genesis chapter 3 talks about now having to work the ground and fight the thorns and weeds. God says that we will eat the "herb" of the field. There are probably many reasons for this, but there are a couple that really make sense to me. One of the things my doctor taught me when I was first learning to regain my health was that man, without any work, becomes very depraved. God's "curse" on man having to work the ground for food was actually a blessing.

The hard work God gave to man kept him from becoming a completely depraved being. In order to grow vegetables man must till the ground and fight weeds and other things that destroy crops. Fruit trees don't need a lot of work once they are planted. The fruits that grew on those trees in the garden were so easy to just pick and eat.

Another reason for the added need for vegetation in our diets is when sin entered the world things were no longer perfect. Now we have the stresses of everyday living that drain our bodies of vital minerals. Vegetation provides needed minerals to give back to the body what stress takes away. Still, even after the fall, the very best diet for us is provided by the creation that God made for us. He gave us fruit-bearing plants, and then He gave us a way to grow vegetation.

Eating our food as close to nature as God has provided for us gives our bodies living food—food that is alive with vitamins, minerals and enzymes. Doesn't it only make sense to fuel living bodies with living food? Our bodies are made up of living cells. These cells are constantly making new cells and can only use what we give them as building materials. Don't we want our living cells to have the very best material possible?

So what happens to these bodies when we try to fuel it with mostly cooked, processed, and denatured food? Even worse is when we feed it mostly food that is not food at all, but things that only mimic food. These things would be the toxic products we put into our bodies, things like soda pop, processed meats, fast foods, and other things that are full of chemicals. If we only stopped long enough to read what is in these products, I am sure we would at least be *hesitant* to go ahead and eat them. Although I know there are skeptics who would still refuse to believe that it is really all that important to shun those junk foods and choose to eat raw, living foods.

Many people have the argument, "If what I am eating is not really food, then why am I still alive? Why do I have energy each day, and why am I still walking around just fine?" I can only say that if we truly knew what was going on in our bodies, we would be shocked into silence. These bodies are working hard every moment at living, and many times living in *spite* of what we are doing daily; certainly not because of it.

When we eat mostly cooked and processed food, the body has to "make do." By that I mean the body takes what it gets and uses it, yes, but it also has to steal from the reserves the body has. If we give the body less than the complete package, which is what we do when we eat food that is dead, then it must borrow (or worse yet, steal) from areas in the body. This is how diseases eventually happen. Some diseases happen early in life and some later.

Every individual is different. There are many factors that come into play when determining the life of each person. Some people just may have more in reserve than others do. Remember the Pottinger cat experiment? That experiment alone explains a lot. Read back over that part in the book again and let it sink in.

How soon in life a person gets an illness or disease also depends on just how toxic a person eats. There are neutral foods that do not give life back to the body, but they also do not steal too much from the body either. Then there are toxic foods that not only are cooked, but have harmful things that the body must neutralize. These foods rob the body greatly.

The foods we have talked about so far in this chapter swing from raw, living foods to toxic, junk foods. Let's say we have three categories of foods that we routinely put into our bodies for fuel...or even just for enjoyment. It really doesn't matter whether we are eating for fuel or for enjoyment; anytime we put something into our body, our body must deal with it. Those three categories of food are: (1) raw, living foods, (2) neutral foods, and (3) toxic, junk foods.

Let's mix this up a little here! I want to talk a bit about the neutral foods first. These foods would be foods that do not add a toxic load to the body, but also do not give the body any real nutrition. They do in some ways "steal" a bit from the body because the body must use some of its reserves to process and to be able to use them for fuel. Remember, the total package must be in the food for the body to truly use it without borrowing or stealing from reserves. The total package cannot be there if the food is cooked because all the enzymes have been destroyed.

At the same time, these foods are not in the same category with the toxic, junk foods because the body does not have to neutralize the toxins or worse, store them away. These neutral foods would be things like baked potatoes, whole-grain breads, whole-grain pastas, brown rice, steamed vegetables, etc. These foods could make up a small percentage of a person's daily diet. If wise choices are made with this small percent a person could stay vital and healthy eating these kinds of foods along with a very high raw diet.

The third category of foods, the toxic and junk food, is food that is not only devoid of enzymes and nutrients but also has things in them that the body must neutralize. These are foods like soda pop, foods with white sugar and white flour, fast foods, etc. The list could go on and on. I think most people will know what foods I am referring to here. These foods force the bodies to not only take from its reserves of enzymes, but also to pull vital minerals from different parts of the body to neutralize the toxic effects they have on the body. The acid in soda pop, for instance, causes the body to pull calcium from the bones to neutralize it before we can deal with passing it through the body. These toxic and junk foods should have no place in a healthy diet.

Now let's get to the good news! Let's talk about those foods God originally created for us. This first category, the raw and living foods, will give the body life. They will not only fuel the body to let us live our daily life, but in some cases they will even pay back deficiencies in our body. How much life is in the food and how easy this food is to digest will determine how much life-giving health these foods will give to the body.

There are some raw foods that are very easy to digest and will give the body much in the way of nutrients and life. Then, there are some raw foods that are hard to digest. The body will use up most of the nutrients that are in the food just to digest that food. Still, the body does not have to borrow from its own reserves to use this food. Then there are even some raw foods, believe it or not, that actually cost the body more than they are worth! In order to gain vitality and health, we need to focus on those foods that give the most to the body.

Let's determine which raw foods we need to maximize in our daily lives and which ones we should minimize. I am not saying we need to be absolutely perfect in our daily lives, but we do need to be aware of what we are routinely eating. It is not enough to just say, "This food is raw, so it is good for me." Let's educate ourselves and learn which foods are best for our body and make sure those make up the majority of our diets.

In order to discuss these different kinds of raw foods and their effects on the body, I am going to put the raw, living foods category in three categories of its own. Let's talk about those categories from the bottom up!

The third category of raw food, the ones that actually cost the body more energy than they are worth would violate that one principle of the "real food" test. You remember... the one that says you must be able to eat an entire meal of this one substance. An example of this would be garlic. Many health advocates claim that this is an amazing healthy thing our body needs daily. I do not think, though, that anyone would want to sit down and eat a whole meal of garlic. The same is true for onion. While some people say that onions are a great health food, they do violate this principle.

There are many things grown by nature, but that does not mean God made them to be food for us. I don't mean that we cannot use them in foods occasionally for flavor, but let's not fool ourselves into thinking they are health-giving foods.

The second category of raw foods are the raw foods that do not cost the body anything to deal with, yet don't really give much back either. These raw foods are those foods that use their own enzymes for processing when we consume them, but really there's not much nutrition left over to give the body building materials to work with. Many people who adhere to a raw food diet would say that a food that has not been cooked above 112 degrees is raw because the enzymes have not been destroyed. While that may be true, it does not mean that those foods are the best foods for us.

For one thing, most of the water in dehydrated foods has been removed so is unavailable for the body to use. These foods can have a place in a healthy diet, and along with the neutral foods, could make up a very small percentage of the daily diet, but they should never take center stage. The majority of our foods need to be the fresh, living fruits and vegetables with a bit of raw nuts and seeds. Now we are ready to talk about the very important first category of raw foods. This category *should* take center stage!

In the first category of raw foods we have those things grown by nature that we do not have to process in any way to thoroughly enjoy. These foods are the complete package; they have everything in them needed to process through the body and also give some back to its reserves. These foods are especially important when the body is in need of healing, which most of our bodies are!

Because these foods are so health giving, we should make them 75–80 percent of our diet in order to stay in good health and even more prominent in our diet when we are already in a state of disease. The body can stay in great health when eating this high raw diet and can heal completely even of chronic, degenerative diseases when special care is taken to give the body the nutrients it needs in the form it needs. We'll talk more about what this kind of diet actually looks like on a day to day basis in a later chapter.

One of the absolute best raw foods we can consume is freshly made fruit and vegetable juices. I realize some people would argue that we are "processing" the fruits and vegetables when we juice them, and that is true. While I know by juicing fruits and vegetables they are no longer in the form God made them, I do believe they should have a prominent place in our daily diets. This is in part because we live in a fallen world where the fruits and vegetables just do not have the high quality of nutrients they should have and also because most of us already have health issues we are dealing with.

Freshly made juices remove the fiber and concentrate the nutritional qualities in fruits and vegetables, giving them to us in a form the body can readily use. Because the fiber has been removed, our body does not have to work to digest them. All the nutrients can be used by the body for healing and for energy.

Freshly made fruit and vegetable juices are very concentrated with vitamins and minerals, so we should treat juices as a complete meal. Never drink juice with a meal; that would be overloading the stomach and would defeat the purpose of the juice. Also, allow plenty of time for the juice to be completely absorbed before you eat a meal. When you drink a juice, take your time sipping, so the body can take full advantage of all the nutrition there.

Since all the fiber has been removed in freshly made juices, we can take in much more nutrients at one time. For instance, you would have a very hard time eating five or six carrots, several leaves of lettuce, a couple of stalks of celery, and an apple. Just chewing all that thoroughly would be exhausting! Juicing it all together, though, concentrates all that wonderful nutrition in a glass and gives our body a much needed break from the hard work of digestion. Since the body does not have to work at digesting, all those nutrients in that glass of juice can go right to work healing and fueling the body.

Because of this very fact, diets rich in freshly made juices are an amazing way to help the body heal from chronic, degenerative diseases. A great book to read on this subject is Dr. Joel Robbins' book, *Juicing for Health*. In it, he not only explains why juicing is the absolute best supplement you can include in your diet, but he also gives many juice recipes. There is even a section at the back of the book on primary nutrients, their use in the body, symptoms of deficiency, and common food sources of that nutrient. I have found this book invaluable and so handy and easy to use.

God has given us an amazing array of fruits, vegetables, nuts, and seeds. It is amusing to me when I hear someone say they would be bored eating a predominately raw diet. I've even heard people say that life would not be any fun! Most of those very people who say that have not even begun to touch the surface of all the different fruits and vegetables God created. There is no better or more refreshing food than the foods God created to not only sustain us, but to keep our bodies in great health.

I think more than anything, people do not know how to not only *include* more raw foods in their diets, but to give them the place of prominence where they are the *focus* of the diet. The thought of making raw fruits and vegetables 75–80 percent of our total diet is an overwhelming and yes, I guess, a boring thought to most people.

This is only because we have been trained to think of food as entertainment instead of fuel for our body. Food should be eaten to give our bodies the energy and vigor we need to have fun and live life and to do the work God has for us to do. Food was not meant to be the *source* of fun.

Up to now, I have talked mainly about the whys of eating mostly raw. Let's talk some now about how to do this and hopefully we'll see how freeing and even fun eating God's original diet plan can truly be.

how to eat
for great health

Try to suspend your beliefs about nutrition for a time while we talk about how to eat for great health. Most of us have a belief system in place when it comes to healthy eating. We believe breakfast is the most important meal of the day and maybe should even be our largest meal. We believe we must have animal protein to build muscle. We also believe we need dairy for strong bones and teeth. None of these things are true.

When I hear someone tell people that breakfast is the most important meal of the day, I think to myself, "Breakfast is the most important meal of the day *to miss.*" Our bodies are in a cleansing time during the hours of four a.m. until noon. That is the time of day our body is taking out the trash. Do you ever notice when you wake up that you have that bad taste in your mouth we sometimes call "morning breath"? That is one sign your body is working on cleansing.

When we head for the kitchen and have something heavy in the morning we stop the body's cleanse cycle; the body must stop that important job of cleansing and begin digesting. How many years could you go around your house without ever taking out the trash? Things would get pretty disgusting after just a short time, wouldn't they? In essence, this is what we are doing when we never let our body complete its cleanse cycle; we are preventing it from taking out the trash.

If we want something to eat in the morning, it should be something very easy to digest; foods that take very little to no digestion like freshly made juice or juicy fruit. Eating light like this will allow the body to continue the cleanse cycle and is actually very satisfying. Once you get used to eating light for breakfast, you may choose to eat nothing at all. One great way to start the morning is having a glass of pure water, squeezing in some fresh lemon juice.

As we move on to another very common false belief we have about nutrition, we should be able to see clearly why this belief does not make sense. When someone tells you that you must have animal protein for strength, do a bit of research and see for yourself what has happened to those countries that eat the most animal protein. Those countries have the highest incidence of cancer. For one thing, animal protein is most always cooked, so it is dead. This will force the body to have to use its own enzymes to process it.

As for the protein in animal products, it is way too high for our bodies. The body cannot use all of the protein in them, so it must store it away. Fruits and vegetables do indeed contain protein. Raw plant protein is in a form the body can readily use and is in much smaller amounts than in animal products, which is a good thing because stored protein ferments in the body and can cause a toxic overload.

Think about this fact. We do most of our growing in the first six months of life. Ideally, we do that growing on human breast milk. Did you know that human breast milk actually has a *lower* percentage of protein than many fruits and vegetables?

Another thought-provoking question is this—where do some of the strongest creatures on earth (bulls, gorillas, apes, etc.) get their nutrition? They get it from the plant kingdom! When you search for truth with an open mind, putting aside long-held beliefs, it is amazing how God shows you His truth. It all begins to make sense.

Another preconceived belief about nutrition is one taught from early childhood. That is that we must have dairy for strong bones and teeth. Where did this idea originate? It originated with dairy farmers. The calcium in dairy is not in a form the body can readily use, especially when the dairy has been pasteurized. There is actually more calcium in many fruits and vegetables than in dairy products; additionally, the calcium in fruits and vegetables is in a form that the body will readily recognize and be able to put to good use. Again, search for the truth. Since government studies have pushed dairy products for "bone health," the instances of osteoporosis have gone way up, not down.

If we have now determined that we should indeed greatly reduce and even eliminate animal protein and dairy, what then should we eat? The answer is fresh fruits, vegetables, nuts, and seeds; the original diet our Creator designed for us. Again, I know at first thought this way of eating sounds boring, and you may think it lacks variety. That is so far from the truth! God made many, many kinds of fruits and vegetables; they just have been pushed from our minds and plates because we have for decades been eating so much in the way of animal products and processed foods. When you think about this, you begin to realize that as we have eaten more animal products and junk foods and less raw fruits and vegetables, we've seen the health of our nation go down measurably.

What if we turn this around? What if we concentrate on eating less processed foods and animal products, and more raw fruits and vegetables? Can you imagine what would happen? I believe we would see the health of people abound. We would see a sharp reduction in cancer rates, heart attacks, strokes, and diabetes, as well as a host of other ailments. Even the mental state of people would be healthier.

It is important to know that our body has a definite cycle which, when followed, helps it to work at its peak performance. We've talked a bit about the cleansing cycle when we were discussing what to have for breakfast. The whole pattern of the body's cycles looks like this: Noon to eight p.m. is the digestive period. Our body's metabolism is set up for digestion. Eight p.m. to four a.m. is the assimilation period. The body is mobilizing nutrients to the cells. Four a.m. to noon is the elimination and cleansing time. The cells are dumping waste products and making and repairing the cells.

It is best to eat in conjunction with the body's cycles. Eating late at night, for instance, causes stress on the body and makes it hard to get good sleep. Sleep is the time the body is assimilating nutrition and getting ready to use it to heal.

At least 75–80 percent of our diet should be raw fruits and vegetables, and we need to eat raw foods at every meal. The more raw foods we have in our diets the better, of course, but there are some rules we need to follow. One of the most important rules is to never overload your stomach. Overeating, no matter how healthy the food is, will cause what food your body cannot use to sit in the stomach and putrefy.

Food combining is another rule we will discuss, although if you are eating a correct diet of mostly raw fruits and vegetables and if you are eliminating animal products, you will not have to worry too much about this. Food combining is important if you have trouble with digestion.

In the transition period of changing the diet to a mostly raw one, people might need to pay close attention to food combining. Food combining is eating only certain categories of food at one meal. For instance, always eat melons alone; never combine them with anything else. This is because melons digest so quickly, much like freshly made juice.

Even with fruits you can divide the categories so as to get the best digestion. Sweet fruits go well together. Bananas and dried fruits are examples of sweet fruits. These go well with celery and lettuce, but do not digest well with acid fruits.

You may combine sweet fruits with sub-acid fruits. These are fruits like apples, grapes, peaches, pears etc. The sub-acid fruits combine well with the acid fruits; those fruits are oranges, pineapples, kiwi, strawberries, etc. You should eat fruits alone and not combined with other foods. An exception to this rule would be apples. Apples go well with anything.

Non-starchy vegetables go well with most any food. Non-starchy vegetables include cauliflower, broccoli, zucchini, cucumbers, peppers, and more. The starchy vegetables are best combined with green salads (no tomatoes) and do not go well with protein. Corn, carrots, pumpkin and potatoes are examples of starchy vegetables. Greens such as lettuce and celery go well with anything.

Proteins are best combined with salads and are especially hard on the digestive system when eaten with starches. Concentrated plant proteins are nuts and seeds. If you do choose to eat animal protein from time to time, be sure to leave off the starch…no potato or bread with that steak! I have heard my doctor say that when you eat a meal of steak and baked potato, it takes nine straight meals of all raw fruits and vegetables just for the body to be able to neutralize that meal.

Okay, I said at the end of chapter five that we would hopefully see how freeing and fun eating God's original diet for us would be. I'm sure by now some people are feeling a bit overwhelmed and do not really see the "fun" or the freedom in this diet! I promise, once you start eating this way you will see the fun and freedom in feeling good all the time with lots of energy and joy through the day.

The freedom comes when you no longer are bound to disease, prescription medication, and the fear of what aging will bring. I also love the freedom I feel *from* the cravings of food that was toxic and heavy to my body. I love being free from feeling that I had to have certain foods in order to have fun. It's so freeing to realize that I am eating to live, not living to eat. Food no longer has the hold on me it once had. The joy and gratitude I feel to God for my healing is worth everything!

The fun is there too! It is so much fun to see my children excelling in sports and having plenty of energy. It's a blast to hear them tell me how much better they perform when they eat raw foods instead of heavy, cooked foods.

It makes me grin from ear to ear to hear that they finally get it!

Imagine how freeing the mornings will be now. You do not have to rush through a breakfast that you really are not even hungry for. Breakfast now is a fruit smoothie, a glass of freshly made fruit or vegetable juice, a nice juicy piece of fruit, or maybe even just a glass of water with freshly squeezed lemon juice. Think how enjoyable your morning devotion and prayer will be with all that extra time! Be sure to keep plenty of fresh fruit on hand so you will always be assured of a simple, fresh breakfast. Also peel and freeze very ripe bananas and put them in freezer bags. Have some of your favorite fruits cut up and frozen, too. Then your morning can be as simple as blending up your favorite fruits and some water or fruit juice into a healthy, beautiful fruit smoothie!

Lunch can be a wonderfully refreshing glass of freshly made vegetable juice; or if you are away from home at lunch time, consider making juices up in advance and freezing them in canning jars. The frozen juice will make a nice cold-pack for fruits or vegetables you may want to take in your lunch for the day. The juice will be thawing through the morning, and by lunchtime will be ready to drink. My husband hurries his frozen juices along by holding them in his hands and letting the heat from his hands thaw the juice.

Sometime after you are sure your juice has absorbed nicely in your body (don't rush it; give your body plenty of time to get the full effect of the juice's nutrients), have some fruit in season or a nice fruit salad. Vegetables and homemade raw dips are also a great thing for lunch, as well as a salad with a variety of vegetables and greens.

Use your imagination! Salads do not have to be just lettuce and tomatoes. There are multitudes of vegetables that you can use to give your salads different tastes and textures. Remember, apples go nicely with anything, so they can be added to give a crunchy, sweet addition to a bed of mixed greens.

Dinner can be much the same as lunches. You can add steamed vegetables, baked potatoes, whole-grain bread, rice, or pastas; or you can keep dinner time all raw by staying with salads and a variety of dehydrated dishes.

The thing to remember is keep your day at least 75–80 percent raw, with the remainder of the food being high-quality whole grains or other foods processed as little as possible.

Keeping the day all raw and only having cooked food for dinner time (being sure to make a salad or some other raw food the main focus of the meal) is an easy way to keep track of making sure you are consuming a very high raw diet.

Give yourself some credit! You have imagination, use it! You know if you decided you wanted to feed your family a totally different kind of ethnic food, you would have to go through a learning time. So give yourself time to adjust to this high raw foods lifestyle.

Learning to eat healthy and changing your diet to predominately raw foods can be fun and exciting when you consider the changes you will witness in your and your family's overall physical and emotional health. Read books about raw foods to educate yourself.

Keep fresh in your mind the reasons *why* you are working so hard to feed yourself and your family nutritious foods. Search out some great raw food recipe books and learn how to prepare a variety of dishes in beautiful and appetizing ways. Find a raw food preparation class. Subscribe to raw food newsletters online. Make it a fun adventure for your whole family!

More than anything—know that you and your whole family are not only going to feel better and more energetic, but as you educate yourself and begin to fully understand how God made our bodies to be in health, you will be living with amazing peace of mind.

eating healthy on the go

I know how busy life can get. It is hard and can sometimes seem impossible to eat healthy with our busy, hurried lives. In this chapter, I want to show you ways to stay with the plan—ideas to keep your family on track even in the busiest of times.

You do not have to resort to fast food to keep your family fed when schedules get crowded and family members are going in many different directions. I know at times it feels like you are rarely home long enough to do laundry and sleep!

One thing I want to say first is … it gets easier as time goes on. The healthier your family members get, the simpler the menus will become. I know for my family, as time goes on, my children seem satisfied with less food and simpler menus. As I mentioned in an earlier chapter, they actually *request* simple things like fruit smoothies or just a few pieces of fruit if they are going to ball games or practices. They have figured out how much better they feel and perform when they eat light and all raw.

I have some very busy, active children still at home—from pre-teen to late teens—and they all agree that they'd rather just have fruit when they are really active. There was a period of transition, of course, when we were getting used to eating this way. It wasn't too long, though, before they felt the difference it makes when they eat simple raw foods.

There are times, especially during the height of basketball season, when we are gone all day and sometimes into the late evening. On days like that, we pack a cooler with a variety of fruits to eat in between games or appointments. We also keep fruit and vegetable juices frozen for days when there is no time for juicing fresh.

Normally we juice fresh every day, and we always juice extra so we have at least a jar or two each day to put into the freezer. Then when we need to take a juice with us, it is there and ready.

If we are going to be gone over the dinner hour also, we cut up vegetables for veggie sandwiches and pack them separately from the whole-grain bread. Sometimes we'll make a few sunflower seed butter sandwiches to take along too. We've even made veggie roll-ups with whole grain tortillas, chopped veggies, homemade raw salsa, and avocados, and then packed them snugly together in a glass dish wrapped in plastic wrap.

There's just never a reason why you should have to resort to unhealthy fast food. Even in a pinch, you can make the healthiest choices possible. If there are really no other options, and you find yourself out and unprepared, you can choose salads at most any restaurant. There's also the choice of a veggie sub sandwich on whole grain bread. It is not the best in nutrition, but is much better than a burger and fries!

When you do let down and make those choices, don't fret! Remember, it's the grand scheme of things that count. The majority of the times, what do you find yourself doing? When you look back over the course of the week, what did you and your family's eating look like? Do some evaluation, and if these times of less than great choices happen infrequently and you see that you are getting better at providing great raw food for your family, then be encouraged!

If, as you honestly think about it, those times are way more frequent than you'd like, then change something! Put some thought into it and see that with a little more planning and ingenuity, you can and will get through the transition time. Before you know it, you and your family will be living a life of healthy eating that just comes naturally, even in the busiest of times.

Life is so much more than eating. I love it that I look forward to the things we are doing each day instead of what we are going to be eating. It's so much fun to grab an ice chest and fill it with God's amazing fast food (fresh fruit!) and run out the door with my children to the next soccer or basketball game.

Always remember...it is *much* more fun eating to live than living to eat!

Examples of foods for those on-the-go times:

fruits

- bananas
- apples
- bags of freshly washed grapes
- cartons of freshly washed strawberries (put these in containers as opposed to baggies; they tend to crush easily)

- oranges (makes the car smell so nice when these are being peeled!)
- cherries

trail mix

These can be made with many variations using nuts, seeds, and dried fruits. Always use organic dried fruits because of the chemical preservatives used in commercially dried fruit

veggies

- carrot sticks
- cucumber slices
- bell pepper strips
- celery sticks
- jicama sticks
- all these can be packed in Ziploc bags

dips for veggies

- spinach dip*
- raw hummus*
- dill miso/tahini dip*
- guacamole*

These dips can be put in several small sealed containers for individual dipping, or if it's "all in the family" and you don't mind double dippers, one family-sized container.

wraps

Use whole-grain tortillas, or for better nutrition, the sprouted grain tortillas found in health food stores. For best nutrition of all—collard greens sliced in half with the center vein removed makes a great wrap. If you are using some of the raw dip recipes for the dressing, you will have an "all raw wrap!"

If you are using tortillas for your wrap, lay a Romaine leaf on it first, to keep them from getting too soggy. Then spread the dip of your choice from the above list, fill with chopped veggies, and roll up. These can be individually wrapped or packed snugly in one large dish and either sealed with a lid or, if the dish is glass, sealed with plastic wrap. These travel nicely for those car trips or all-day outings.

sandwiches

The directions for veggie sandwiches are pretty much the same as for the wraps. For great nutrition use sprouted grain breads. Put the condiment of choice on the bread. (There are great raw mayo recipes and other sandwich dressing recipes available in many raw food preparation books—or use a non dairy mayo found in health food stores.) Then put the bread in baggies separate from the veggies. In sealed containers or plastic bags put greens, sliced avocados, cucumber slices, sliced tomatoes, sprouts, red pepper strips, etc.

We make up separate sacks of these for each child because everyone wants a different condiment or different veggies on their sandwich. When it's time to pull out the sandwiches and eat, everyone finds the sack with their name and puts their individual veggies on their bread. My children love this take-along.

You can also use any raw nut butter with a raw honey or make your own pureed fruit for a nut butter and honey or nut butter and jelly sandwich. For good nutrition, make sure to use whole-grain bread. For great nutrition, use the sprouted grain breads.

frozen juices

It's great to juice extra each time you are juicing fruit or vegetable juices and freeze the extra up in jars. This makes it so convenient to grab a jar for each one in your family and put them in the ice chest with all the fruits and veggies.

Or if you are going to be consuming them right away, just find a box small enough for them to fit in snugly, and once you are all on your way in the car, have everyone keep their juice handy. They can "work on" thawing them by holding them in their hands.

It is also a good idea to take spoons along so you can chop them up for faster thawing, or just eat the juice as a slushy. Always remember to take a small box along to contain all the jars after they are empty so they are not rolling around on the floor of the car!

smoothies

It is fun to have a take along smoothie cup with a straw and lid for each member of the family. You can make a plethora of different kinds of smoothies to serve up in your take-along cups right before you head out the door. Everyone loves having their own cup to sip on in the car.

These smoothies can be many variations of fresh fruits with frozen bananas and ice, or for extra nutrition, make them "green" smoothies. These are smoothies that are 60 percent fruit and 40 percent greens. I will include some smoothie recipes in the recipe section of this book, but once you make a few, you'll come up with your own favorites.

You can probably see now how easy it is to stay the course even in the busiest of times. With a little planning and creativity, you'll be so pleased that your family can eat healthy and still be active doing all the things you all love to do. You are not giving up anything! You are on the road to a life of great health and lots of energy to be the busy family you love to be!

*These recipes will be included in the recipe section of this book.

what to expect in the beginning —
cleaning up the diet and detoxing

When you and your family first begin the transition to eating more raw foods, you may feel overwhelmed. At first, any change in life can seem to knock everything off track. Give yourself and your family some time to get used to this way of eating. If you have been used to filling much of your diets with convenient pre-packaged foods, or using lots of fast foods to get you through busy days, then things may be a bit harder at first.

If on the other hand, you have tried to pay attention to nutrition and have been using fresh fruits and vegetables in your daily diet, things should be easier. You do have to remember, though, that just including fresh fruits and vegetables in your diet versus making them the main focus of your day can be a difference of night and day.

I believe we can fool ourselves into thinking that we are eating healthy. We may say we eat "lots" of fruits and vegetables, when in reality they have just been a garnish that we have added to our mostly cooked and/or processed food diet. It is important that we are honest with ourselves. Look hard at what you and your family are consuming on a daily basis and decide for yourself if you are truly eating an abundance of fresh, raw fruits and vegetables.

I remember one time a lady I had not seen in several years approached me at a curriculum fair. She heard about my cancer diagnosis and knew that I had chosen to stay away from the traditional medical route. She told me she had just been diagnosed with cancer, and she wanted to hear what I had done to get well.

When I started telling her about nutrition and its role in healing cancer, she stopped me and said, "Oh, I already eat healthy."

I simply asked her if she ate at least 75–80 percent raw fruits and vegetables.

She answered, "No, but we eat lean meats, whole grains, and no white flour or sugar."

It seemed a wall went up at that point, and I couldn't get her to see that while that sounds wonderful compared to what the standard American is eating, it is not the nutrition the body needs to get healthy and stay that way. I remember telling her that I thought I ate healthy too, until I really started understanding what the body needs for health.

Again, we have *got* to understand what foods the body needs for health, in addition to what things we need to keep out of our diet. So before we go on with talking about what to expect when we change our diets to at least 75–80 percent raw, take a minute to evaluate what you and your family have been eating on a consistent basis. I don't just mean from time to time eating raw fruits and veggies, but what does your diet honestly look like?

Once you get a picture of the things in your diet you

abounding health naturally

need to change, it'll be nice to know what you can expect when you focus on eating mostly raw. The body will definitely go through some changes. It will be cleaning house, repairing and rebuilding because now it will have the energy and quality tools with which to do those jobs.

It will seem at first that your body is sick; maybe even worse off than before you cleaned up your diet and added high quality raw foods. What is actually happening, though, is the body is going through a detoxification phase. You will hear it referred to as *detoxing*.

I hesitate to use that word because it seems at times it is overused! The fact is, when your body has been fed junk food for so long, (or maybe it has been food that is not particularly junk, but would still be qualified as "lifeless") there is a lot of work to be done.

Sometimes this work is not too pleasant. Just remember that there is probably an abundance of trash to be taken out. If you can know what to expect from the beginning, you will be better prepared for what is happening and even be grateful for how you see your body responding to the improved nutrition it is receiving.

Some signs the body may be detoxing can be things like fatigue, cold, or flulike symptoms, a bad taste in the mouth, soreness in the muscles, headaches, mucus, congestion, nausea, dark urine, depression, blemishes, fever, diarrhea, stomachache, irritability, etc.

Getting more rest and extra sleep, drinking lots of water, spending time in the sunshine and fresh air can help the detoxification process. Doing enemas and colonics can also help facilitate the process.

You may also find as you make the transition to more raw foods, that your emotions become "raw." It could be that these are emotions you may have buried with that box of chocolates or bag of potato chips and they are now coming to the surface for you to deal with. As your body gets healthier and healthier, you will be better able to deal with these emotions, but in the beginning, look for ways to get through these times.

Take time to go for a walk every day. Getting outdoors for a brisk walk can do wonders to lift depression. Take a warm bath, read a good book. Find creative ways to help this cleansing process; don't suppress it.

Believe it or not, this can be a great time to organize and clean house! When you have the physical energy to do so, tackle those cluttered drawers and closets. It is amazing how energized you can feel when you know you are clearing out areas of your home. It almost feels that all that "stuck energy" is released.

Lastly, but most important of all—pray and spend time with the Lord. He is the One we should have turned to anyway in those emotional times instead of that chocolate bar! Memorize portions of His Word and meditate on them. Psalm 119 is a great passage to begin with; it is full of reasons why we as believers should love His law. "Oh how I love thy law! It is my meditation all the day"(Psalm 119:97 KJV).

God promises success to those who will meditate on His Word. "This book of the law shall not depart out of thy mouth; but thou shalt meditate therein day and night, that thou mayest observe to do according to all that is written therein: for then thou shalt make thy way prosperous, and then thou shalt have good success" (Joshua 1:8 KJV).

As you study God's Word, find verses that especially

speak to *your* heart. Write those on three by five cards to carry with you through the day. Memorize them and then meditate upon them as you make them part of your life. It is amazing what we can accomplish when God's Word is not only on our lips, but deep within our hearts. Let Him help you make this time of transitioning into a healthier, *rawer* diet an adventure—even on those days when you know you *must* be cleansing!

organic versus conventionally grown

One big concern most people have when they think about eating more raw foods is thinking they absolutely *must* buy all organic fruits and vegetables. Most people are worried that there is no way they can afford the expense of buying everything organic. I have even heard people say that they won't change and start eating mostly raw foods *because* they know they will have to buy all organic and they cannot afford it. The funny thing is these same people are eating the standard American diet, seemingly not worried at all about how it is processed!

Wouldn't it be so much better to concentrate on including more raw fruits and vegetables, then as you are able, buy as many of them as you can organic. Do not use the excuse that you cannot afford it. If you cannot afford organic, then buy conventionally grown.

There are ways around this problem. One is to grow as much as you can yourself. Another good way to buy pesticide free produce is to regularly go to farmers' markets. Ask the farmers at the stands whether their fruits and veggies are organic. Many times they are, but the farmer cannot put that organic label on his produce because it has not been "certified" organic. From what I understand, it takes years to get that stamp of organic certification.

Keep your eyes open. I find many times organic produce is as cheap as or sometimes even cheaper than conventionally grown. I have been amazed as I watch people automatically pick up grapes that are conventionally grown, when right down the row are organically grown grapes that are the same price.

Usually (not always) the organic produce not only tastes better, but is higher in nutrition because the farmers pay attention to the way they farm the land. For the most part, they take better care of it than the big commercial farms do.

When you cannot buy organic, just soak the produce you are getting ready to prepare for consumption in a sink half-filled with water and an ounce of apple cider vinegar for fifteen minutes or so. This will help to cut the waxes and pesticides on the fruits and/or vegetables.

There are some fruits and vegetables that are sprayed more and/or absorb more of the pesticides than others. Use this list to make decisions on what is best to buy organic.

dirty dozen (highest residues)

1. Peaches
2. Apples
3. Sweet bell peppers
4. Celery
5. Nectarines
6. Strawberries

7. Cherries

8. Pears

9. Grapes (imported)

10. Spinach

11. Lettuce

12. Potatoes

cleanest twelve (lowest residues)

1. Onions

2. Avocados

3. Sweet corn (frozen)

4. Pineapples

5. Mangoes

6. Asparagus

7. Sweet peas (frozen)

8. Kiwi Fruit

9. Bananas

10. Cabbage

11. Broccoli

12. Papayas

After all is said and done, and we have done the best we can, we must trust that God will protect and know that we can rest in Him.

When I was first diagnosed with cancer and I was just beginning to understand the important role diet plays in health, I worried much about wanting to buy everything I could organic. I freaked out about a lot of things then and lived in so much fear.

One lady told me "Sharon, if I cannot buy organic, I just wash the produce really well and pray over it. I pray for God to put back in the food what He intended to be there and to take away what He did not." I think that is awesome!

So, do the best you can with what you have. Do not make excuses, but also do not fear. Trust God to take care and provide what you cannot.

Live your new health conscious life to the fullest, knowing God will honor your endeavors to take care of the body He has given you.

healing from disease

In this chapter, I will give more details about actually healing from disease. There are things in this chapter I have already addressed, but I want to go over them again in a somewhat different way. I hope by doing this the truths of how the body heals will really sink in. I know there are those people who will be reading this book who feel defeated and find themselves despairing. I am praying for this chapter, as well as the whole book to bring much encouragement and hope.

Most of this book has dealt with changing the way we eat so we do not have to worry about illness and disease. We want to be well and stay well. I remember listening to Phillip Day's CD, *Cancer, the Winnable War,* when I was first diagnosed. At first, all I could hear was how we could stay well and never have to fear the disease. I don't know why, but I felt defeated at first, thinking, "Well, I already *have* cancer, so now what do I do?"

I do not know if everyone feels this way, but I know I so desperately needed to hear someone tell me that it didn't matter; I needed someone to believe for me, that I could and would heal of this disease, and that I would not have to ever fear cancer again.

In the beginning, I went to medical doctors when I had problems with my health. As I said in an earlier chapter, I had clue after clue that things were not right in my body. Early in our marriage, I had infertility problems. When I had exploratory surgery to find the problem, the doctor was surprised to see so much endometriosis in someone so young. He felt he had to remove one ovary and one tube.

From my early twenties, I had problems with fibroid tumors. The first I knew about was found in yet another surgery for infertility. These were removed, and I went home to heal. For years I lived with a growth behind my right ear. It caused severe headaches, and at times I *lived* on over the counter medication to ease the pain. I finally went to a doctor who diagnosed it as a fibroid tumor of the parotid gland. This was the *only* doctor (until I went to Dr. Robbins after I was diagnosed with cancer) who actually addressed nutrition. He did not talk about fresh, raw, and living foods; he didn't have a sound teaching on nutrition, but it was clear somehow he knew nutrition played a part in health. I look back now and see that he wanted to avoid surgery if possible. The pain finally got so bad that I asked him to go ahead and schedule surgery to remove the tumor.

My mind did not comprehend that poor nutrition had anything to do with my health problems. After the birth of our sixth child, I had four miscarriages. Finally, a few years after the last miscarriage, I could feel a large mass in my abdomen. I again went to a doctor who diagnosed it as a large fibroid tumor and recommended a hysterectomy. Still… my eyes were not opened; still nothing clicked with me that there was something wrong with the way I was feeding my body.

Not until I was diagnosed with stage three breast cancer did I begin to question the route I was taking with my health. Now it was life and death, and now it was a diagnosis that I would have to live with the rest of my life...which according to the medical authorities I had seen, might not be very long; certainly not as long as I wanted to live...not long enough to raise my children and to enjoy my grandchildren. Now, even though I was terrified, I was determined to find another answer.

After two surgeries to remove the lump and after seeing an oncologist and hearing his gloom and doom statements about my life, I insisted my surgeon remove the port-a-cath she put in during surgery. She didn't ask if I wanted to do chemo...she said I *had* to do chemo. I made the decision to remove myself from the traditional medical doctors and find another way. I decided very quickly that I did not want to do chemo or radiation; I did not want to live always looking for cancer to come back. I knew I was through with the constant medical tests. I wanted to be free of cancer, to be healthy and strong, and to never look back.

It is strange that for so long I thought I would always have this dark thinking about myself. I thought I would always think of myself with the shaded view of having had cancer. Now, at times, it almost seems like it happened to someone else. I remember when I watched Dr. Lorraine Day's video, *Cancer Doesn't Scare Me Anymore*, thinking what a blessing it would be to feel that way. Well, it is a blessing because I do feel that way! Cancer does not scare me anymore!

As I read books and listened to recorded teachings and seminars over and over, it finally sunk in; yes, I could heal from disease, even this awful disease of cancer. You can have that confidence too. It takes more than just doing what someone else says to do, though. You must be determined to understand for yourself how your body works. Do not just sit back and let others, no matter how good their intentions are, tell you what you need to do. Yes, seek out a nutritional doctor who can walk you through getting your body back to true health, but at the same time begin your self-education. There are a multitude of great books to read and wonderful audios available. Be careful to listen with your heart of discernment. Make sure the things you are reading and listening to are sound. Ask God to give you "hearing ears and seeing eyes" to see and hear the truth.

There is much on the Internet you can explore and learn about raw foods and their role in health. You'll learn about enzymes and how cooking foods kill those vital things our body needs. So many of the raw food sites, though, are very new age in nature, and don't give credit where credit due. Just be mindful, though, that just because the information is presented in a wrong way does not make all the information wrong. Be careful what you buy into, but also be careful about what advice you throw away.

God created raw foods. Remember it was His idea in the beginning. Just because someone may pervert the teaching of nutrition does not mean we need to throw out the good with the bad. Study—learn and apply what you know to be true. Have confidence God can heal your body when you begin to take care of it in the way He designed.

I remember when I was first learning about raw foods and the role they play in the body's health, I worried that for some reason it wouldn't work for me. As I studied and read, I was beginning to understand true nutrition and how and why cancer develops in the body. Still, I had this mental block, causing me to wonder if it would actually work in *my* body.

I remember sharing this with a precious friend of mine. This friend knew how fearful I was and called me every morning for many days in a row to spend time in prayer with me. She was ecstatic that I had chosen to heal through nutrition instead of going with the ravages of chemotherapy and radiation.

This one particular morning when I told her how afraid I was that it wouldn't work for me, she said, "Now, Sharon, why wouldn't it work for you? You see how the body heals, and there's no reason it won't work for your body. It's not like you are a lizard and everyone else is human!"

I think that was the first great laugh I had in many weeks! She not only gave me the gift of laughter at that moment, but she also gave me an insight into the faulty thinking I had. I was not thinking truth. God made our bodies to function a certain way. He created them to live on live foods and to heal naturally when we treat our bodies correctly.

I clung to that funny statement my friend made for a long time. Every time I would start to doubt, I remembered that indeed I was not a lizard! I was human just like everyone else. Many, many people found healing when they gave their bodies whole, raw nutrition, the food God designed for the body to function at its best. Reading and hearing testimonies of people who changed their diets and healed their bodies naturally is a great way to turn the doubting into believing.

So with that thought in mind, if you are suffering

from a disease, *know*—beyond a shadow of a doubt—God made your body to be in health. He made your body an amazing creation after His own image. It is only through abuse and neglect that we fall into diseases. Make the determination right away to educate yourself and get going full force on giving your body what it needs to heal.

It is important to surround yourself with people who can and will believe for you when you are weak and doubting. I remember one dear friend in particular who gave me the gift of "believing for me." One day, when I was having an extremely hard time believing for myself, she spoke words of encouragement to me. I will never forget what she said to me. She looked me straight in the eyes, smiled, and said, "It's okay, Sharon. We are believing *for* you. We are praying and claiming God's healing *for* you."

It takes time to be strong enough to believe for yourself that God will use nutrition and faith in Him to heal your body, especially when we are trained to think differently. We must retrain our thinking; we must search God's Word for verses of healing and keep them fresh in our minds. We have to learn what is true about health and nutrition; what is true about how God made our bodies. We need to make it a habit to think and dwell on truth while we are being responsible and relearning how to feed our bodies.

I had another friend who would help me to determine if the thoughts I was having were valid thoughts. She would always direct me to a certain Scripture verse, "Finally, brethren, whatsoever things are true, whatsoever things are honest, whatsoever things are just, whatsoever things are pure, whatsoever things are lovely, whatsoever things are of good report; if there be any virtue, and if there be any praise, think on these things" (Philippians 4:8 KJV).

When I was depressed and found myself dwelling on statements doctors or other people had made, she would take me through the "thought test." I remember one time in particular saying to her, "What if what the oncologist said *is* true?"

She responded, "Well is it a good report? No, it is not, so it fails the test!"

I gradually learned to get through each and every dark thought that way...if it failed the Philippians 4:8 "thought test," then it got thrown out!

It takes time to get through those dark thoughts we put upon ourselves, but we can do it. If God commands we are to "think on these things," then we can know for certain that we can retrain our thinking to always dwell on whatsoever things are true, honest, just, pure, lovely, and of good report! It is amazing the healing work our body can accomplish when our thoughts are lined up with these truths.

It takes time to get yourself to the place that you are strong enough to be around people who question and doubt. Much the same as it takes time to tame and train your own thoughts; it takes time to be able to dismiss the comments of others. So, as much as possible, limit who you are around to people you can trust to be positive about your healing. Of course, you cannot avoid all negative people, and there will be times you just have to toughen up. You will eventually be strong enough emotionally to fend off any comments made, but for a while, protect yourself.

I can remember when someone's comments about my having cancer or even just a comment about cancer in general would leave me shaking with fear. I would hold up long enough to get home, and then I'd break down in tears. I knew who I could call upon, though, to help me build myself back up! I had my husband, who believed *for* me…beyond a shadow of a doubt…that I would be well and strong and completely free of cancer soon. I also had a handful of friends I knew I could count on to believe for me. I look back now and see what an incredible army of people God put in my life to hold me up through those dark days.

I am going to talk more in another chapter about attitude and its importance in our health, but I just felt I needed to touch lightly on getting the right frame of mind from the start if you are battling a disease. You can literally "burn up" all the good nutrition you put into your body if you are lying awake at night worrying about your fate!

Once you have determined that you know God made your body to be in health, and you know that God made great food from the very beginning to fuel these bodies for a lifetime, get started! Find a doctor who can help you understand what you need to do and why.

I am very prejudiced…I feel I had the absolute best doctor, and I am so grateful God gave me direction to this doctor. My doctor ran some tests to see where my body was deficient and what I needed to supplement to beat the cancer as quickly as possible. He told me "once you have cancer, it is like a race to get ahead of it." (Praise God, it is a race that can be won!) He taught me about nutrition and why my body was in the state it was.

It was eye opening to understand that the body really had to work hard to even stay alive with the way I had fueled it for so many years. My liver was having to do things it was not designed to do and my digestion was terrible, so what food I was eating was not being assimilated, and on and on.

When you are already in the state of disease, it is not always enough to just start eating all raw foods. You need guidance to get through it safely and effectively. There is much to learn to help the body to heal quickly.

When my mother was first diagnosed with cancer of the bladder, the doctors removed her bladder, and she had to live with a bag the rest of her life. I had not been through my bout with cancer at that time, so I didn't know there was another answer to cancer...I didn't know the real answer to cancer.

Later, when the cancer returned in another location in her body, I asked her to try nutrition instead of going through all the chemo the doctors wanted her to do. She and my dad agreed that, yes, that is what they wanted to do. They had seen me heal from cancer just a year or so prior to that, so they were confident. My mom immediately started eating all raw foods. She had an appointment to see my doctor, Dr. Joel Robbins, but she didn't wait...she began eating all raw right away.

What we did not know was my mother had an ulcer, and her stomach could not tolerate all the raw food. She began throwing up blood. I put a call through to call Dr. Robbins. He knew what was happening and helped us through that time until he could see her.

In addition to the ulcer, my mother was not digesting her food well, so her body was not receiving the nutrition it needed even from the raw food. The digestive system needed a break. It needed to totally rest to be able to heal. So how could the digestive system totally rest and the body still receive nutrition? The answer...juicing!

Freshly made fruit and vegetable juices work wonders in getting live nutrition right to your body without the body having to work for it. We are able to get an amazing amount of live vitamins and minerals through freshly made juices. Since all the fiber has been removed, the digestive system can rest *and heal.*

My mother, much like I did, started her journey in healing cancer with a month-long juice diet. For four weeks she consumed only freshly made fruit and vegetable juices. At the end of four weeks, when we added back fresh and raw fruits and vegetables, the body was able to digest and use them.

Juices are still a big part of my and my family's life. We juice daily to make sure we are getting plenty of vitamins and minerals in a form that is easy for the body to use.

A glass of freshly made juice is the absolute best multivitamin you could ever find. Be sure you make vegetable juices much more prominent than fruit juices. Fruit juices are very cleansing and full of enzymes, but especially if you are in the state of disease, vegetable juices are more important to consume. Vegetable juices are rebuilding. They are full of minerals, which most bodies are very lacking in.

I have already touched some on the fact that you need to educate yourself, but I still want to say it again and to explain in a bit more detail the "why." Do not just take what someone says and do it, hoping for the best.

What others tell you may be great advice. It may be the absolute truth, but unless you own it, unless you make it part of who you are, things will not change for long. You may take the advice and completely heal your body, but it won't be long before you go back to eating and living the life that sickened your body in the first place.

I have known several people who used nutrition to heal from cancer, only to succumb to cancer later down the road. The reason always boiled down to the fact that they did not make the information their own information. They did not own what they knew was truth. They used nutrition much the same as someone would use medicine...just to get well and be rid of illness and disease.

In order to be truly successful at regaining complete health, you must have that picture in mind—complete health. Don't just have that limited vision of healing from disease. For one thing, when you do that, you are keeping disease in your focus. We must focus on what we want, and that is health.

When the focus is on healing from a disease, the mind tends to stay very narrow. We get a tunnel vision, and we keep the disease in a prominent place in our minds. We do not want the disease in our body *or our minds!* Remember we are to be retraining our minds to think on "these things"! So, again, instead of dwelling on getting rid of disease, concentrate fully on gaining great health.

At first, this seems impossible. Many of us are so accustomed to thinking of the negative anyway, but especially after a shocking diagnosis it is very difficult to begin to think true thoughts. It is incredibly hard because most of us have looked to doctors all of our lives as the ones who have the answers for health. When these doctors have told us grim news and our future looks pretty bleak in their eyes, our thoughts are dark. We have to remind ourselves over and over, that for the most part, doctors do not have the answer for health. Their answers lie in dealing with disease. This is their area of expertise. They have been trained in how to deal with diseases.

I love a statement Phillip Day makes on his recording, *Cancer, the Winnable War*. He was commenting on many doctors' answers for cancer, but this comment he made would apply for most every disease. He said, "When all you have is a hammer, everything looks like a nail." The things doctors have to offer people who are sick and diseased are prescription medications, pharmaceutical drugs, surgery, etc. That's all they have—the "hammer" they have been trained to use. Doctors are not trained to teach people how to live in health or how to regain health. They teach you how to live with a disease.

Please be sure I am not trashing doctors. I just want you to understand where they are coming from. When you fully understand that, you can put what advice they have given and the predictions they have made for your life in proper perspective.

Once you gain perspective on what you have been told, you can change your thoughts. You can know that you have not been told the complete truth. You have only been told what someone else *thinks*. There is only one true God, and it is His truth we want.

Here's the job you have to do. Focus on truth. Think correct thoughts. Run every thought through the "thought test" of Philippians 4:8.

Now, learn true nutrition. Learn how God made our body to be in health. Find a doctor who understands true nutrition to help you through this time. Teach yourself and your families how to eat and to use food for nutrition—whole, live nutrition for a whole live body.

Read all you can on the subject and use discernment. Pray and ask God for wisdom to show you what is truth regarding nutrition. Not everything out there is truth, and we need His wisdom to give us discernment. Make no one your authority; only God has that place in our lives. It is our responsibility; our job to take care of this temple God has given us. Do not pass that God-given mandate on to *anyone* else.

Determine that you will live your life in health. Don't make food of any kind your god. Our God is the Creator who designed our bodies *and* the food to fuel our bodies. We can live our whole life in health. None of us know how long we will live; God alone determines the length of our life. We *can*, however, live the life we have with vitality and enthusiasm!

I am convinced that we hold in our hands what the quality of our life will be. Through apathy and ignorance, we can live with illness and disease; or through responsibility and knowledge we can live in joy and health. You have to determine for yourself what kind of life you truly want. Remember, though, the choices you make not only affect you, they will affect all those God places in your life's path.

I want to share some scripture I used to meditate on during those months I was learning that I *could* and *would* beat cancer. These passages hold a special place in my heart. My husband used to read these passages and many others to me day and night! The sound of his voice reading God's truths gave me peace and confidence.

Study these passages and find others in God's Word that especially speak to your heart. Meditate on them day and night to give you strength and confidence…and most of all His complete and overwhelming peace.

> He that dwelleth in the secret place of the Most High shall abide under the shadow of the Almighty.
>
> I will say of the Lord, He is my refuge and my fortress: my God; in Him will I trust.
>
> Surely He shall deliver thee from the snare of the fowler, and from the noisome pestilence.
>
> He will cover thee with his feathers, and under His wings shall thou trust: His truth shall be thy shield and buckler.
>
> Thou shalt not be afraid for the terror by night; nor for the arrow that flieth by day;
>
> Nor for the pestilence that walketh in darkness; nor for the destruction that wasteth at noonday.
>
> A thousand shall fall at thy side, and ten thousand at thy right hand; but it shall not come nigh thee.
>
> Only with thine eyes shalt thou behold and see the reward of the wicked.
>
> Because thou hast made the Lord, which is my refuge, even the Most High thy habitation;
>
> There shall no evil befall thee, neither shall any plague come nigh thy dwelling.
>
> For He shall give His angels charge over thee, to keep thee in all thy ways.
>
> They shall bear thee up in their hands, lest thou dash thy foot against a stone.
>
> Thou shalt tread upon the lion and adder: the

young lion and the dragon shalt thou trample under feet.

Because he hath set his love upon me, therefore will I deliver him: I will set him on high, because he hath known my name.

He shall call upon me, and I will answer him: I will be with him in trouble; I will deliver him and honor him.

With long life will I satisfy him and show him my salvation.

Psalm 91 (KJV)

I will extol thee, O Lord; for thou hast lifted me up, and hast not made my foes to rejoice over me.

O Lord my God, I cried unto thee, and thou hast healed me.

O Lord, thou hast brought up my soul from the grave: thou hast kept me alive, that I should not go down to the pit.

Sing unto the Lord, O ye saints of His, and give thanks at the remembrance of His holiness.

For His anger endures but a moment; in His favor is life: weeping may endure for a night, but joy cometh in the morning.

And in my prosperity I said, I shall never be moved.

Lord, by thy favor thou hast made my mountain to stand strong: thou didst hide thy face, and I was troubled.

I cried to thee, O Lord; and unto the Lord I made supplication.

What profit is there in my blood, when I go down to the pit? Shall the dust praise thee? Shall it declare thy truth?

Hear, O Lord, and have mercy upon me: Lord, be thou my helper.

Thou hast turned for me my mourning into dancing: thou hast put off my sackcloth, and girded me with gladness;

To the end that my glory may sing praise to thee, and not be silent. O Lord my God, I will give thanks unto thee forever.

Psalm 30 (kjv)

For I know the plans I have for you, declares the Lord, plans to prosper you and not to harm you, plans to give you hope and a future.

Jeremiah 29:11 (niv)

If thou wilt diligently hearken to the voice of the Lord thy God, and wilt do that which is right in His sight, and wilt give ear to His commandments, and keep all His statutes, I will put none of these diseases upon thee, which I have brought upon the Egyptians: for I am the Lord that healeth thee.

Exodus 15:26 (kjv)

Bless the Lord, O my soul, and forget not all His benefits: Who forgiveth all thine iniquities; who healeth all thy diseases: Who redeemeth thy life from destruction: who crowneth thee with lovingkindness and tender mercies: Who satisfieth thy mouth with good things; so that thy youth is renewed like the eagles.

Psalm 103:2–5 (kjv)

He is despised and rejected of men; a man of sorrows, and acquainted with grief: and we hid as it were our faces from Him; He was despised, and we esteemed Him not. Surely He hath borne our griefs, and carried our sorrows: yet we did esteem Him stricken, smitten of God, and afflicted. But He was wounded for our transgressions; He was bruised for our iniquities: the chastisement of our peace was upon Him; and with His stripes we are healed.

Isaiah 53:3–5 (KJV)

Heal me, O Lord and I shall be healed; save me and I shall be saved: for thou art my praise.

Jeremiah 17:14 (KJV)

Thou wilt keep him in perfect peace, whose mind is stayed on thee: because he trusteth in thee.

Isaiah 26:3 (KJV)

I will bless the Lord at all times: His praise shall continually be in my mouth. My soul shall make her boast in the Lord: the humble shall hear thereof, and be glad. O magnify the Lord with me, and let us exalt His name together. I sought the Lord, and He heard me, and delivered me from all my fears. They looked unto Him, and were lightened: and their faces were not ashamed. This poor man cried, and the Lord heard him, and saved him out of all his troubles. The angel of the Lord encampeth round about them that fear Him, and delivereth them. O taste and see that the Lord is good: blessed is the man that trusteth in Him. O fear the Lord, ye His saints: for there is no want to them that fear Him. The young lions do lack, and suffer hunger: but they that seek the Lord shall not want any good thing. Come, ye children, hearken unto me: I will teach you the fear of the Lord. What man is he that desireth life, and loveth many days, that he may see good? Keep thy tongue from evil, and

> thy lips from speaking guile. Depart from evil, and do good; seek peace, and pursue it. The eyes of the Lord are upon the righteous, and His ears are open unto their cry. The face of the Lord is against them that do evil, to cut off the remembrance of them from the earth. The righteous cry, and the Lord heareth, and delivereth them out of all their troubles. The Lord is nigh unto them that are of a broken heart; and saveth such as be of a contrite spirit. Many are the afflictions of the righteous: but the Lord delivereth him out of them all. He keepeth all his bones: not one of them is broken. Evil shall slay the wicked: and they that hate the righteous shall be desolate. The Lord redeemeth the soul of His servants: and none of them that trust in Him shall be desolate.
>
> Psalm 34 (KJV)

Reading, memorizing, and meditating on Scripture will have a powerful effect on our minds. As we cleanse our minds with God's Word, He will bless us with the ability to act upon the truths He gives us.

Jesus Christ gave Himself for us, His church "that He might sanctify and cleanse it with the washing of water by the Word" (Ephesians 5:26 KJV). What an amazing thought, "The washing of water by the Word"! We desperately need our minds to be clean through His Word so we will be able to live the lives He has for us.

the best of the best

God created His best for us in the beginning at creation. Before sin entered the world we had the best of everything. Nutrition in the garden of Eden was the best of the best. All the fruit was perfectly ripe and sweet. All the nutrient value God intended to be in the food was there, readily available to the body for use in building new healthy cells and to keep the body supplied with fuel for energy. The body was kept in tip top condition. The world was perfect; no stress, no worries, perfect food, no pollution, fresh air and sunshine, perfect relationships... all was well.

Then sin came on the scene. From then on, things were not the same. As time has gone by, the nutrient levels in our food may not keep up with what we need. Even organic raw foods are lacking in the value God intended them to have. Don't get me wrong, we should still be eating mostly or all raw foods, but there are times when we need more. This is all the more true because of the toll stress takes on our bodies. The world we live in is far from the perfect place God created. We can still live our lives in health... it just takes more work to do so.

In our current times, I believe the best of the best includes freshly juiced fruits and vegetables, green smoothies, sprouts, and wheatgrass juice. I am sure there are more things that many health conscious people consider "super foods," but these are the four groups I will focus on in this chapter. These are the things that everyone can include in their daily lives to stay disease-free, energetic and healthy for life.

In the matter of juicing, I hear people argue that God did not create the fruits and vegetables "juiced," and that is true. It is also true that God made fruits and vegetables in the beginning to be much more nutrient packed than they are now. God also did not create this world to be in the disarray it is in. So when we juice, we are making up for the fact that most fruits and vegetables are not the nutrition packed creation God originally created them to be. Also we are using juices to supplement the body and fuel it to be able to function more healthfully in this stress-ridden world.

For juicing you will of course need a juicer. Try to get a good machine that will last you a long time and is easy to use and clean up. I don't like the typical machines you find in most department stores because they are usually not well made and won't stand the test of truly using them over a long period of time. Also, most of these machines are ones that operate on centrifugal force. They spin, so they actually spin oxygen into the juice and cause the enzymes in the fruits and vegetables to oxidize at a faster rate. We are using juices to get an amazing amount of vitamins and minerals in a way our body can readily use, so we want to juice in the most efficient way possible to preserve all these things our bodies are so hungry for!

We use a masticating (also known as a grinder-strainer) juicer. We have used a Champion juicer for several years and like it for its efficiency, durability, and ease of cleanup. When you juice every day, sometimes several times a day, you definitely want a juicer that is not only durable, but easy to use.

In juicing, we are able to pay back deficiencies and supply our bodies with the best multi-vitamin available. You cannot always know what is in vitamin supplements you buy in the stores, but you can know that when you drink a glass of freshly juiced carrots and greens, you are getting just that—all the vitamins and minerals that are in carrots and greens, concentrated!

Freshly made juices are the best way to get live nutrition into your body efficiently.

In *Juicing for Health*, Dr. Joel Robbins states that he has worked with patients who do not like fruits and vegetables, so he tells them to drink at least two glasses of fresh fruit and vegetable juices a day. He states that what happens is usually "just short of a miracle." These patients begin to feel better and their tastes and cravings begin to change. They eventually come to the point where fresh, raw fruits and vegetables are more attractive to them .

When I was first diagnosed with breast cancer, Dr. Robbins put me on a four-week juice diet. My diet consisted of nothing but freshly made vegetable and fruit juices for that whole month. This allowed the digestive system in my body to rest so it could heal. At the same time, I was getting amazing nutrition packed in a glass. I drank more vegetable juices than fruit and had somewhere between a half to three-fourths of a gallon of juice daily.

If you only have time for one juice a day, make it a vegetable juice. Especially when ill, the body is in great need of minerals. Vegetables are more important than fruit in this area. Many people say don't even juice fruit, just juice vegetables. We do juice some fruit in the mornings, but if we don't have time, I don't feel bad skipping fruit juice.

However, I refuse to let my family skip the daily vegetable juice! I am adamant that this is important to our health. I hope by strictly sticking with vegetable juices every day I am implanting a great habit in my children's lives that they will never give up and will pass on to their children.

Juices can be made from practically any fruit or vegetable. I love to juice greens, partly because I think greens are an amazing healing force for the body, but I also just love the taste of greens. I like to juice a lemon and some apple with many different kinds of greens, including dandelion greens! Our basic vegetable juice that we all have daily consists mostly of carrots. We add different greens to a base of carrot juice. Most days we use romaine lettuce or kale, but some days we like to switch to parsley, beets, and cucumber. We almost always add celery and a bit of apple to our carrot juice.

We also like to make "green" smoothies several times a week. A green smoothie consists of 60 percent fruit and 40 percent greens. You can have lots of variety with green smoothies because there are many wonderful combinations. They fit nicely into a busy life because they are fast and easy to make and the cleanup is quick. If you have frozen fruit all cut up and in the freezer ready for making smoothies at a moment's notice, they are the ultimate fast food!

We really like our Vita-Mix blender for making all our smoothies, and it is especially helpful with green smoothies. You can either add ice or use frozen fruit to make the smoothie cold and thick. Frozen bananas are especially good in these green drinks, as well as in most smoothies. The high speed blenders, like the Vita-Mix, work wonderfully in blending all the greens smoothly with the fruit and do a great job in turning out a nice creamy drink. When you include green smoothies daily in your high raw diet, and at the same time eliminate processed foods, I think you'll be amazed with how quickly you begin to see results in your health.

I will include some favorite green smoothie ideas in the recipe section of this book, but I don't think it will be long before you are coming up with your own family's favorites!

Sprouts are another powerhouse of nutrition. Sprouting is also fun, economical and a relatively easy way to supercharge your diet. Sprouting is the process of soaking, rinsing, and draining seeds until they germinate, or sprout. Growing your own sprouts adds life and, depending on which kinds of sprouts you grow, zest to your family's diet.

Sprouts are baby plants in their prime. Because they are in their prime, their vitamin and mineral content is much greater than at any other point in their growth. They have rapidly multiplying enzymes, vitamins, minerals, and even protein! The B vitamins alone increase by 300 to 1,500 percent in only three to six days! Sprouts are a fresh, living food and because they are grown right in your kitchen, you can have a fresh harvest year-round. They are a great way to add an amazing amount of nutrition to your salads, sandwiches, and wraps.

The last "best of the best" I want to talk about is probably my favorite; and believe me, it is not my favorite because of its taste! I have a soft spot for wheatgrass for many reasons, not the least of which is it is so much fun to grow. Juicing and experiencing its powerful life force is almost a side benefit!

Wheatgrass is a variety of grass that comes from the shoots of the wheat berry. It is widely acknowledged as a powerful super food in nature. Wheatgrass juice is quickly becoming one of the most popular supplements used by health conscious people.

Wheatgrass juice is often called "liquid sunshine" as it contains over 70 percent chlorophyll. Because it is absorbed into the bloodstream almost immediately, this juice can be a potent blood cleanser in the body. Chlorophyll is recognized not only as a cleanser, but also as a rebuilder and a neutralizer of toxins. One ounce of wheatgrass juice is equal to two and a half pounds of vegetables in nutritional value. Wheatgrass juice is truly an amazing source of great nutrition, and you only need a small "shot" of it daily to appreciate what it does for your body.

When someone asks me what wheatgrass juice tastes like, the only thing I can say is "green"! When people are visiting our home and they see wheatgrass growing in the kitchen, they are always intrigued. One reason is it is so pretty to see trays and trays of green life growing inside the home, but they also wonder what I do with it. When I tell them that everyone in our family has a shot of wheatgrass juice every morning, many times they want to taste a bit—and a "bit" is all you need at one time. Two ounces of wheatgrass juice is as much as the body can absorb and use at a time. To get the full benefit, be sure to drink it on an empty stomach.

If you are interested in trying wheatgrass juice, try to find a health food store in your area that sells shots of it. It is fairly expensive to buy this way, especially if you begin to drink it daily. For quite some time, I visited a local smoothie shop just to get a shot of wheatgrass juice daily. I really wanted to grow my own, but I thought it was probably too tricky for me, as I have never had much of a green thumb! I got a couple of books and a video and began to educate myself.

When I realized how cheaply you can grow trays of wheatgrass, and also because I was determined I wanted this amazing source of nutrition for my whole family, I took the plunge and began to grow it in my kitchen. It wasn't long before I saw how incredibly easy it is to grow. It is very satisfying too because it grows so quickly. You can see it coming to life right before your eyes! I have recently turned over our wheat grass production to our twelve-year-old son. He is doing a wonderful job of tending it and keeping our whole family supplied with plenty of wheatgrass juice.

In juicing wheatgrass, you will need to have a juicer that is able to do the job efficiently. The Champion juicer will not juice wheatgrass, but you can purchase inexpensive juicers that are made just for wheatgrass. We bought one recommended by the master wheatgrass grower at Hippocrates Institute. It is a single-auger manual juicer, and I was amazed how efficient it is in getting the juice out of the grass. This juicer is called "The Healthy Juicer" and also comes in an electric model.

Don't let any of these things overwhelm you. Pick one or two of those things you feel you can do and go for it. I recommend you start drinking freshly made vegetables juices right away because you will see results quickly.

Those results will encourage you to stick with your new healthy lifestyle.

Be sure to include your whole family in all the preparations and fun! All of my children juice, make smoothies, and take part in every facet of our raw diet. Our youngest child has been juicing since he was seven years old. I remember he stood on a booster chair to be able to push the vegetables through the juicer! Educate your children while you are educating yourselves. Our children not only know the "how to" in preparing nutritious food, but they also know the "why."

live life in motion!

It is a bit funny to have to actually say "live life in motion" because most people are hurrying through every day of their lives. Life certainly *seems* to have a lot of motion. Moving should be the last thing we'd have to be reminded to do. The kind of motion I am talking about, though, is not the stressful day to day way we are living our lives. Running from one activity to another is not necessarily what I am referring to, although it *can* be, if we are doing it with the right motivation.

When I talk about living life in motion, I mean to fully be a part of everything you do. Don't just go through the motions; really put your all into what you do. Enjoy the world God has made for us. Don't let day after day go by without getting outside, truly thanking God for fresh air and sunshine and for the ability to enjoy those things with the healthy body He has created for you. No matter what physical condition you find yourself in, you can thank God for the health you *do* have.

It would be easy to just say, "Okay, for good health, you must get exercise, fresh air, sunshine, breathe in, breathe out, one, two, three, and four!" However, in some ways, that just adds more stress to an already stressful life.

Don't get me wrong, it is vitally important that we include fresh air, sunshine, and exercise in our daily lives. We must move our bodies to keep everything flowing.

The lymph system does not have a pump of its own; we need to have daily exercise to keep it healthy. The sun is also a vital part of our health program. We need the vitamin D it gives, and the life-giving energy it supplies. Breathing in the fresh outdoor air is crucial to not only our physical health, but our emotional health as well. Our homes and work places have become so airtight, that I've heard our indoor air is more polluted than the outdoor air.

So, yes, while all these are very important to our health, wouldn't it be nice to just *enjoy* all these things as a part of the way you are living your life instead of *making* yourself include them because you know you need them to be healthy?

It seems when we get it in our heads that we must do these things, it takes all the fun and joy out of them. These things become part of our "to do" list, instead of part of the vibrant way we are living our lives. Maybe this is because our lives have become so *still*. Instead of living our lives, we have almost become spectators. We sit at the computer, we sit in front of the television, our children are sitting with their iPods, texting with phones, playing their handheld video games, etc. We have become a culture of people who have to be told *to move*.

We have also become a culture of *indoor people*. It is rare to see a family out enjoying a friendly ball game, having a picnic, or working in the yard together. Most families spend their days and evenings indoors, with each family member doing their own thing. There was a time when most family members spent much of their time outdoors. The day would start early with chores to do to keep the family farm and household going. From the young child through the grandparents, there was something important for each family member to accomplish to keep things running smoothly. Work was hard and no one had to be told to get in some exercise and fresh air. It was something that came naturally. Even with all the hard work they had to do, they still had time for family and friends. People then enjoyed life with family members and their neighbors.

In modern times, even with all the labor and time-saving devices we have, we are busier than ever. Instead of moving our bodies, though, we are pushing buttons and doing very little physical work. Those who do have a job that entails physical labor don't get much satisfaction out of it. They work to get the job done and then go home and crash in front of the television. Bedtime gets pushed back until the wee hours of the morning in the name of getting more done; still we go to bed without the satisfaction of truly giving our body a good day's work.

I do not pretend to know what the answer is to this life of inactive stress. I know we cannot go back to times with no computers or cell phones, but how nice it would be if we could get control over them, instead of these things controlling our lives. We have traded a life of active productiveness *with* our families, a life where you didn't need to worry about exercise and fresh air because those things were *lived,* for a life of stress— rushing to accomplish tasks without family togetherness. We have no real time for fellowship with friends and neighbors. We are living a life where we have to be told to exercise every day and to get outside and get some fresh air and sunshine.

If you do not have an occupation you truly enjoy, find a way to change that. Either love the job you are doing, or do the job you love. We have been tricked into thinking we must work for the most money possible, when in fact, if you are doing something you are passionate about, the money is secondary. Of course we need money to live in this world, but when you are doing something for others with their welfare in mind, you won't have to worry about where the money will come from to pay the bills. You can always tell when someone is working just for the money, can't you? From the cashier at the grocery store to the serviceman repairing your washing machine, it is evident if that person truly loves helping you or is just waiting for the clock to say it is time to go home. In general, which person do you think is healthier? Which person do you think is going to be more successful in life? It is the one who is joyfully serving others in their profession; the one who truly loves the job they are doing.

As for exercise, don't just schedule it in for the sake of exercise. Find something that you truly look forward to doing. Find ways to involve people you love being with. Get tasks accomplished while you are exercising. You don't have to lift weights to build your body. There should be plenty of chores that need doing that will also build muscle and tone your body. Of course if you love lifting weights and working out, by all means, do so! The point is to find activities that you can truly enjoy and that you can be consistent in doing. Even taking a nice long walk with your spouse or child will do much more than just begin to tone your body…it will tone up relationships too. So, who in this case do you think is healthier? The person who squeezes in some time at the gym, rushing from the gym to work, or the person who landscapes his yard with his family, the person who is designing projects to better his life and his family's life? The person who naturally exercises his body while truly living his life in motion is healthy in body and soul.

Take time to be in the great outdoors, feeling free to breathe in the fresh air and letting your skin soak up the sunshine. We actually have become a nation of people who are afraid of the sunshine. Before we will go outside or let our children out, we slather on the sunscreen. Is it any wonder we are seeing more people who are deficient in vitamin D? The sun is not our enemy; it is not the sun that is causing an increase every year in skin cancers.

Skin cancer has been on the rise even more since we have been pushing the sunscreen. The lack of nutrients available in our body is a big factor in skin cancer, of course, but we are doing our skin no good by slathering on the chemicals. We do further damage by blocking the sunshine's supply of vitamin D to our bodies. We have actually caused more diseases and ill health since we have been warning people to stay out of the sun and to guard against the sun with sunscreen. Again, we are trying to solve the problem without taking responsibility, and we are only creating more of what we are trying to avoid.

Stop and think about how you are living your life. Are you truly living your life in motion? Are you giving it your all and not just getting through the days? Why do we want good health anyway? If we are just going through the motions each day, why do we need good health? We should desire good health so we *can* live our lives in motion and give to our family and friends the gift of ourselves, truly putting all we have into each moment.

Don't for a second think that I am saying exercise is not important. Exercise is very important, but it loses much of the value for your body when you let stress take over and you don't enjoy the time you spend in exercise. The same holds true for fresh air and sunshine; enjoy the time you spend outdoors. Don't let the cares of everyday life rob you of wonderful times you could spend with those people God has placed in your life.

a merry heart does good

As incredibly important as I believe nutrition is, I know that a proper attitude is an even more important factor in our health. Proverbs 17:22 says, "A merry heart does good like medicine, but a broken spirit dries the bones."

There are many scriptures that allude to the role certain attitudes play in our health. God made our body and fit it with our spirit and soul. They all go together. How we respond to the things that happen to us in life will largely determine how well our body fares when things come along to derail our plans.

It's easy to be happy when all goes as planned. We can sing, smile, and skip along in life when things go our way. It's those times when we feel sideswiped, those events that catch us off guard and send our plans sinking that work to reveal the true character in us. My husband loves the quote, "God is not nearly as concerned about *what* you go through, as He is in *how* you go through it." He takes every chance he can to remind our children of this!

God's Word shows us clearly that our thoughts will influence our whole body. Proverbs 23:7 says, "For as he thinks in his heart, so is he ..." *What* we think about and even *how* we think will determine not only our personality and character, but will in large part determine the health of our body.

In his audio teaching, *Attitudes and Health,* Dr. Joel Robbins says, "Our physical body can and does reflect our thoughts and attitudes—scientific evidence bears this out." And, "Our body can speak to us through our physical ailments. It can inform us of wrong attitudes and thought patterns we are harboring and hiding which are not just creating physical discomfort, but robbing us of much joy, peace and fulfillment in all areas of life."

In thinking about this statement, I realized that I can be very grateful for any physical ailment in my life. Through any illness and even through grave diseases we can know that God is working to perfect us. God made our bodies so perfectly matched with our spirit and soul that we cannot harbor wrong thoughts and attitudes without them directly affecting our body. If we are wise, when we are suffering from any ailment, we will look deep inside and see if there are wrong thoughts and attitudes that have become a way of life. These wrong thoughts and attitudes, if left undetected, not only rob us of physical health, but rob us of the joy God intended for us to have in our lives.

Even if we *could* stay healthy while living with bad attitudes, we are not experiencing the joy we could have in life. So many times we are so focused on how our body feels we are not paying close attention to what is going on with our spirit. When something goes wrong with our body, *then* we stop and pay attention; most of time, though, we are paying attention to the wrong thing.

We are looking for ways to "fix" our body without thinking of what is going on with our thoughts and attitudes. While I am convinced that God holds us responsible for what we put into our body in the way we feed it,

I also know He holds us responsible for those thoughts we allow to live in our minds. Those thoughts are the very things that will form attitudes and actions if we do not change the process quickly.

God says, in 2 Corinthians 10:5 "...bringing into captivity every thought to the obedience of Christ." We are commanded to take captive every thought that does not fall into line with the teachings of Jesus Christ. And how can we know what thoughts those are? God gave us a test for all thoughts. In Philippians 4:8, Scripture says, "Finally, brethren, whatsoever things are true, whatsoever things are noble, whatsoever things are just, whatsoever things are pure, whatsoever things are lovely, whatsoever things are of good report, if there is any virtue and if there is anything praiseworthy—meditate on these things."

Any thought that violates *any part* of that test gets taken captive. That thought gets thrown out. The quicker you take it captive and throw it out, the less chance it has of infecting your spirit. I had a dear, sweet friend who made an amazing analogy when I shared this principle with her. She struggled night and day to get control of fearful thoughts. One day she said, "You know, Sharon, I was thinking of it like a cave. When you first walk into a cave, it would be easy to turn around, head for the light, and walk out; but the further you let yourself wander into that cave, following the twists and turns, the cave gets darker and darker, and it is harder and harder to find your way back out."

I have often thought of that analogy over the last couple of years. How easy it is to capture those wrong thoughts, if when you realize you are thinking them, you turn around right away and head for the light. There's the hard part, though; recognizing wrong thoughts quickly. It takes practice, but you know…practice makes perfect! Start practicing right away.

Many times I have been deep in despair, and it is hours or sometimes even days before I realize that I have not obeyed this command. I have allowed myself to wander deep into the cave and it takes much strength and determination to find my way back out again.

Test every thought against Philippians 4:8. It really is a wonderfully freeing thing when you know, for certain, that a thought is either a God honoring thought, or not. You can know right away if a thought passes *every* point of the test. If it doesn't, what do you do? You take it captive. You do not let it have any place in your mind or heart. The more you practice this, the better you get at it, and the quicker you recognize wrong thought patterns. It is awesome when one day comes and you realize you are standing just outside the doorway to the cave. You catch that wrong thought before it even gets started, and you turn and run the other way!

What an amazing, loving Creator to have so tied our bodies, minds, and spirits together. How kind He is to get our attention that something is not right, that we are not living in the joy He intended for us. No matter what, we can be grateful to Him for allowing our bodies to experience the things it needs to go through in order for our spirits and minds to be free. God wants our minds to be completely free of fearful, agonizing thoughts, and of angry, bitter thoughts.

A wonderful book, *How to Resolve Seven Deadly Stresses* says, "If stressful thoughts are allowed to go from your mind to your heart, they will become a part of your belief system and impair your body's resistance, allowing sickness and disease" (16). It is certainly true that as a person "thinketh in his heart, so is he."

Different emotions damage the body in different ways. No one would argue that a person who is red-in-the-face-angry and then suddenly has a fatal heart attack was directly affected by his anger. Other emotions are a bit harder to trace, but when you examine your thoughts closely, you can definitely see a correlation. For example, Scripture says that, "A sound heart is the life of the flesh; but envy the rottenness of the bones" (Proverbs 14:30). There are studies that show how long held envy will actually cause the bones to deteriorate. It should be no surprise, when you consider this, that osteoporosis is more prevalent in women than in men. Could this be because women, in general, have more of a problem with envy than men do?

As women, we are trained from an early age to want to look like movie stars and models. Even if we do not have a problem with envying how another woman looks, we still "wish" for things that are not ours. For instance, we may envy another woman's relationship with her husband, another person's ability to keep a wonderfully tidy home, and the list could go on and on. The important thing to remember with envy is we are comparing ourselves to someone else. Scripture addresses this action as "not wise."

2 Corinthians tells us, "...but they measuring themselves by themselves, and comparing themselves among themselves, are not wise" (2 Corinthians 10:12 KJV). Our only role model should be the Lord Jesus Himself. There

is never any good reason to compare ourselves with another person.

God instructs us in His Word to "keep your heart with all diligence; for out of it are the issues of life" (Proverbs 4:23 KJV).

We are to guard our hearts against wrong thoughts and emotions. Remember, if wrong thoughts are allowed to go to your heart, that is when they affect your belief system, and as a result will affect your health. In order to guard our heart, we must guard our thoughts. An emotion must start with a thought. As you ask God to give you eyes to see and ears to hear, you will learn to catch those thoughts before they reach your heart and become part of your emotions and belief system.

Keep in mind, it is much harder to get out of that cave if you have been wondering around in there for a long time than it is to turn around and run from the cave before you even enter it!

Examine your heart, thoughts, and emotions. See what is honoring to God and those things that are failing the test of Philippians 4:8. Begin to rebuild the walls of your heart with God's Word. Strengthen your resolve to think and dwell on only those things that *do* pass the test and begin to live the life that God planned all along for us. Live a life of faith in Him with joy, gratitude, and giving to others.

faith in god and service to others

There is no doubt that God takes notice of those who have great faith in Him. Jesus proclaimed to more than one person in Scripture, "Your faith has made you whole" and, "Your faith has saved you." Even today, there are testimonies of those being healed just through their faith in Him. While we don't always know the surrounding circumstances of those divine healings, we know they happen. God in His mercy and grace does choose to heal, at times, on faith alone. Only He knows a person's heart and motives and He alone is worthy to do His work.

I believe faith in God is more than just prayers of asking for healing, protection, and abundance. Faith in God is shown through the living out of His promises. Having faith in God means in part that, we know that what He says is true *is indeed true,* and we are determined to live our lives in accordance with His Word and His plan. We have faith that His commandments are for our benefit and if we truly love Him, we will keep His commandments. We have faith that He is the master designer, and He knows how we should be feeding our body, the thoughts we should be thinking, and the actions we should be taking. We have faith to follow His plan.

Faith in God means we know without a doubt that He hears us when we cry out to Him. We know He hears our prayers. God actually designed us to have a continual conversation with Him. We are instructed in Scripture to meditate on His Word day and night and to pray without ceasing. When we have this fellowship with God our whole body, soul, and spirit are in harmony with Him. When we are in harmony with Him, we will experience His life-giving energy, wisdom, and knowledge.

When we live our life the way God planned—living out our faith in Him through the way we choose to live our life, the way we choose to take care of our body and the things we allow in our minds—we will have a peace that will begin to develop an inner make up that is needed for great health. In His Word, God promises this to those who will live by faith, "It will be health to your navel and marrow to your bones."

Sometimes, though, it is hard to have faith for yourself. When we are ill or weak, we may not have the strength to believe for our own healing. It is easy to doubt and waver when we are experiencing fear and uncertainty about our future. These are the times when God uses the faith and prayer of others. God shows many instances in Scripture where it was the faith of others God used to heal the sick. In Matthew 9, the Bible speaks of four men who had faith for the healing of the man sick of the palsy. They acted on their faith and brought the man to Jesus to be healed. The same is true of the centurion's servant in Matthew chapter 8. The servant was healed because of the faith of the centurion. Jesus told the mother in Matthew 15 when she was asking for healing for her daughter that she had great faith and her daughter was made whole from that very hour.

I experienced personally the faith of friends. When I

abounding health naturally

was struggling with the fear of cancer, I had friends who believed for me. Many times during those hard days and nights I was humbled, yet so encouraged, to have friends who came to me telling me they believed God for my healing. These were steadfast friends who never wavered in their belief that God wanted me well. When I was uncertain of my future, when I didn't know for sure that God was going to heal me, these friends stood strong in their prayers and fasting for me and continually encouraged me to help me build my faith. I do not take lightly any more the statement, "I will pray for you." Those words hold power, and when spoken to someone who may be wavering in their faith, hold much hope.

To experience God's healing should give us a new purpose in life. Our life is meant to glorify God, and when we can testify of His healing power, we have a mighty witness for Him. To be healed is to be brought to a strength and health that will allow us to do a great work that God has planned for us. God wants us to demonstrate His strength and glory to all those in our paths. He wants us to use our lives to bring others first to the saving knowledge of our Lord Jesus. He also wants us to build up the body of Christ. A great way to do that is to help people understand how to live out their lives in health.

That is what I pray this book will be to all who read it. I pray first and foremost that this book will point readers to our Lord. Secondly, I pray those who read this will begin to understand our personal role in our health. I pray God will use the information in this book to open many eyes, and that this could be a beginning of your self-education.

Ask God to lead you and to direct your path to health.

Then, do not be afraid to do those things you know you need to do. Do the hard thing—change your life. You will not be sorry.

menu ideas and recipes

Over the last five years, I have received many questions about health and healing from disease. Many of these questions center on how to fix meals that will be tasty and interesting. It seems when people think of eating mostly raw fruits and vegetables, all they can think of are carrot sticks and celery stalks. They are quite sure most husbands and teenagers will never go for meal after meal of that!

Once you get started on the path of eating mostly or all raw foods, you will find there are ways to prepare foods for taste and variety, yet still keep the vital nutrients intact. To get you started, I will give some suggestions for breakfast, lunch, and dinner menus with some recipes included at the end of the chapter. I strongly encourage you to keep breakfast very light with only fruit or fruit juice, or nothing at all; the breakfast menus will be *very* simple! The lunch suggestions will also be simple and all raw. I will give two dinner suggestions; one will be for those who want to eat all raw and the other for those who want a high raw diet with some wholesome cooked foods at dinner.

breakfast

Pure, warm water with freshly squeezed lemon, and/or one to two ounces of wheatgrass juice can be followed by melons or freshly juiced fruit juice*, or fresh fruit in season (make sure this is juicy fruit, waiting until after noon before consuming bananas or other dense, sweet fruits).

lunch

Vegetable juice* (usually consisting of carrots, greens, apples, etc.). Wait thirty minutes or so, and then have: fruit salad or several pieces of fruit, or vegetable salad with a variety of greens and other garden vegetables, or vegetable sticks with dip*, or apple and celery slices with raw nut butters, or a green smoothie.* Sometime before dinner, it would be great to get in another carrot or green vegetable juice!

dinner

For the all-raw diet, tossed green salads* with a variety of raw dressings.*

With the salad, it is nice to have:

- dehydrated breads*or
- dehydrated crackers* with raw dips*
- raw "pastas"* with raw sauce* or
- raw soups*
- or you could always have another green smoothie* for dinner!

For the high-raw diet: always make a large tossed salad or other raw vegetable dishes your main focus, then include one of the following:

- baked potatoes
- whole-grain pastas
- whole-grain rice
- seasoned oven broiled potatoes
- oven-baked sweet potatoes
- veggie sandwiches on whole-grain breads
- lightly steamed vegetables
- vegetable soups

In this section of ideas for daily living, please remember that these are only a few ideas. You will come up with many more once you get the hang of it and let your own creative juices kick in!

recipes
vegetable juices
carrot-celery juice

6 carrots, scrubbed, with the ends removed
2 stalks of celery
1 apple, sliced

Juice all ingredients through the Champion juicer, juicing celery last.

green juice

3 kale leaves
1/2 bunch parsley
1/2 bunch cilantro
1 celery stalk
1/2 of a cucumber, quartered
1 green apple, sliced
1 lemon, peeled and quartered

Juice all ingredients through the Champion juicer.

fruit juices

apple-lemon juice

6 apples, sliced
1 lemon, peeled and quartered

Juice through the Champion juicer.

orange-pineapple juice

4 oranges, peeled and quartered
1/4 pineapple, peeled and quartered

Juice through the Champion juicer.

apple-pineapple-celery

4 apples, sliced
1/2 pineapple, peeled and quartered
1 celery stalk

Juice all through the Champion juicer.

dressings and dips

guacamole

2 avocados
Juice of one lime or lemon
1 Tbsp Braggs Liquid Aminos

Cut apart avocados and scoop out the flesh (save the pit). Mash avocados with the lime or lemon juice and the Braggs Liquid Aminos. Place pit in the center of the guacamole to help retard discoloration.

spinach dip

4 cups spinach
1/2 cup raw tahini
Juice of one lemon
1/2 tsp sea salt
1/2 tsp dried dill
1 small avocado, peeled (optional)

Blend all in food processor until smooth.

hummus

1 cup peeled and chopped zucchini
3 1/2 Tbsp lemon juice
1 Tbsp olive oil
4 cloves garlic
1 tsp paprika
1 tsp sea salt
1/4 tsp ground cumin
Pinch of cayenne pepper
1/2 cup raw tahini

1/3 cup sesame seeds, soaked for 4 hours, rinsed and drained.

Combine everything except tahini and sesame seeds in high-speed blender, such as a Vita-Mix, and blend until smooth. Add the tahini and sesame seeds and process until creamy.

lemon tahini dressing

4 Tbsp Raw Tahini
4 Tbsp Lemon Juice
2 Tbsp Water
2 Tbsp Braggs Liquid Aminos

Blend all until smooth

tahini-dill-miso dressing

1/2 cup raw tahini
1 Tbsp miso
Juice of 1/2 lemon
1 tsp dill

Add water slowly while blending until smooth and creamy

green smoothies
blueberry/spinach smoothie

2 cups spinach
2 cups frozen blueberries
2 frozen bananas
1 cup water

Blend all in high speed blender, such as a Vita-Mix, until smooth

kale-pineapple smoothie

- 2 cups pineapple chunks
- 4 kale leaves, stems removed
- 3 frozen bananas
- 1 cup water

Blend all in high speed blender, such as a Vita-Mix, until smooth

green/papaya smoothie

- 2–3 cups of greens (your choice)
- 2 cups papaya
- 2 oranges

Blend in Vita-Mix Blender until smooth

raw pasta

Cut the ends off each zucchini squash. Use a vegetable peeler to slice long thin strips from a zucchini squash. You can also use a vegetable spiralizer or a mandolin slicer to make long thin strips. Use these strips for a bed of pasta.

raw sauce for pasta

marinara sauce

- 1 1/2 cups tomatoes, chopped
- 1 date, pitted
- 1 tsp dried oregano
- 1/2 tsp fresh rosemary
- 1 Tbsp lemon juice
- 1/3 cup olive oil

2 tsp sea salt

Blend all in Vita-Mix blender until smooth and spoon over "pasta" noodles.

raw soups

miso/vegetable soup

1 Tbsp miso
1/2 Tbsp raw almond butter
1 cup hot water
1/4 cup chopped vegetables
1 chopped scallion

Let vegetables steep in hot water and then blend in miso and raw almond butter with a fork.

creamy tomato soup

3 large tomatoes
1 cup raw almond milk
1 ripe avocado
1/2 cup fresh basil
1/4 cup fresh oregano
1 tsp sea salt
1/4 tsp cumin
1 tsp lemon juice
Pinch of ground black pepper
Pinch of cayenne pepper

Combine all ingredients in blender and process until smooth. (If you let the Vita-Mix run for a bit, the soup will become warm…be careful to not let it actually get hot!)

salads

spinach/strawberry salad

Baby spinach
Fresh strawberries, stems removed and sliced

Place strawberries on top of a bed of baby spinach and pour dressing over.

Dressing:
    2 Tbsp raw honey
    1/4 cup olive oil
    Juice of one lemon
    1/4 cup water
    1/4 of a red onion
    1 clove garlic
    5 strawberries, stems removed

Blend all in blender until creamy.

fiesta salad

    4 cups chopped romaine lettuce
    2 cups fresh or frozen corn
    1/4 cup chopped red pepper
    1/2 cup chopped scallion
    1/4 cup chopped cilantro
    Sliced raw olives

Dressing:
    2 Tbsp lemon juice
    1/4 cup olive oil
    1 Tbsp Braggs Liquid Aminos or Nama Shoyu
    1/2 tsp ground cumin

Pinch of cayenne pepper

Blend together and toss over salad ingredients

grecian salad

4 tomatoes, chopped
2 cucumbers, chopped
1 red bell pepper, chopped
1/2 red onion, chopped
1/2 cup sliced raw olives

Dressing:
2 Tbsp olive oil
2 Tbsp lemon juice
1 clove garlic, minced

Blend together and toss over salad ingredients

dehydrated bread and crackers
sprouted seed bread sticks

Soak for 6 hours, then rinse and drain:
1/2 cup sesame seeds
1/2 cup sunflower seeds
1/2 cup pumpkin seeds
Soak 1/2 cup flaxseeds in 1 cup of water for 4 hours.
   Do not drain; flaxseeds will soak up the water.
1/2 cup sunflower seeds, unsoaked
1 large celery stalk, chopped
3 Tbsp drinking water
1 green onion, chopped
1/2 tsp sea salt
1 clove garlic, minced

1/4 cup parsley, chopped
1 1/2 tsp dulse flakes
3 Tbsp ground flaxseeds

Place the un-soaked sunflower seeds in a food processor and grind into a fine powder. Transfer to another bowl and set aside. Combine the celery, water, green onion, salt, and garlic in the food processor and process until smooth. Add parsley and dulse flakes and pulse just to mix; leave flecks of parsley showing. Add the rinsed and drained seeds to the processor and pulse into a coarse meal. Transfer to a large bowl. Add the soaked flaxseeds and mix well.

Sprinkle the ground flaxseeds and the ground sunflower seeds over the mixture and knead well to make smooth dough. Allow dough to sit for 20 minutes. Form into bread sticks and place on a dehydrator tray lined with a teflex sheet. Form these sticks fairly flat and have them spaced evenly shaped on the tray.

Dehydrate for 8 hours at 112 degrees. Turn the breadsticks over on to the mesh tray and remove the teflex sheets. Dehydrate another 8 hours, or until the breadsticks are completely dry and crisp.

fiesta flax crackers

Soak for 4 hours: 1 cup sunflower seeds
 1 cup sesame seeds

Rinse and drain.
 Soak 1/2 cup flaxseeds in 1 cup water for 4 hours. Do not drain; flaxseeds will soak up the water.

- 1 bunch (1 1/2 cups) cilantro
- The juice of 2 limes
- 2 tsp sea salt
- 1 tsp cumin
- Pinch of cayenne pepper
- 1 jalapeno pepper with seeds removed

Blend cilantro, lime juice, sea salt, cumin, cayenne pepper, and jalapeno in food processor. Add all the seeds and blend well. Spread mixture onto 2 dehydrator trays lined with teflex sheets. Dehydrate at 105 degrees for 8 hours, then turn crackers over and peel off the teflex sheets. Continue to dehydrate on mesh trays for another 4–6 hours, or until crispy.

afterword

Through much of this book, I encourage you to educate yourself in the matter of health. Because it can be confusing to know where to start in this area, I am including a list of some of my favorite materials I listened to and read to help me in understanding what the body needs and how it works to stay in health. I hope you find these materials helpful to you in your quest for God's truth.

resources

Eating for Health and Wellness, a CD set by Dr. Joel Robbins, DC, ND, MD

Health through Nutrition, a CD set by Dr. Joel Robbins, DC, ND, MD

Juicing for Health, a book and CD set by Dr. Joel Robbins, DC, ND, MD

Attitudes and Health, a CD set by Dr. Joel Robbins, DC, ND, MD

Great News about Cancer in the Twenty-first Century, by Steven Ranson

Cancer, Why We're Still Dying to Know the Truth by Phillip Day

Cancer, the Winnable War, CD by Phillip Day

Health Wars, by Phillip Day

How to Resolve Seven Deadly Stresses, published by Institute in Basic Life Principles

Fresh Vegetable and Fruit Juices, by Dr. N.W. Walker

Diet and Salad, by Dr. N.W. Walker

Become Younger, by Dr. N.W. Walker

e|LIVE

listen|imagine|view|experience

AUDIO BOOK DOWNLOAD INCLUDED WITH THIS BOOK!

In your hands you hold a complete digital entertainment package. In addition to the paper version, you receive a free download of the audio version of this book. Simply use the code listed below when visiting our website. Once downloaded to your computer, you can listen to the book through your computer's speakers, burn it to an audio CD or save the file to your portable music device (such as Apple's popular iPod) and listen on the go!

How to get your free audio book digital download:

1. Visit www.tatepublishing.com and click on the e|LIVE logo on the home page.
2. Enter the following coupon code:
   2c3d-1885-e5f5-4706-c968-926a-3255-4a21
3. Download the audio book from your e|LIVE digital locker and begin enjoying your new digital entertainment package today!